# GUT INSTINCTS

A Journey to Radical Healing,
Inner Knowing & Rewriting the Rules

Jennifer Juniper

Copyright © 2025 Jennifer Juniper
Gut Instincts – A Journey to Radical Healing, Inner Knowing & Rewriting the Rules

ALL RIGHTS RESERVED. No part of this book may be reproduced or transmitted in any form or by any means, electronic, mechanical, photocopying, recording, or by any information storage or retrieval system, for public or private use without prior written permission of the author, except in the case of brief quotations embodied in articles and reviews.

eBook ISBN: 978-1-965761-63-2
Paperback ISBN: 978-1-965761-64-9
Hardcover ISBN: 978-1-965761-65-6
Ingram Spark: ISBN: 978-1-965761-66-3
Library of Congress Control Number: 2025919773

Cover Design: MA Rehman
Interior Design: Marigold2k
Publisher: Spotlight Publishing House™
https://spotlightpublishinghouse.com


Connect:
https://JenJuniper.com

My interest in *Gut Instincts* is a result of being a caregiver. I am attracted to books about life principles in action. Procuring survival skills as an advocate for overcoming chronic illness is a philosophy that parallels my own, and I was looking for a witness.

Juniper's writing style is witty and conversational in content. It is backed up by reflective action steps available to any reader willing to address unresolved trauma. She comes clean on the page, modeling victory over vulnerability in a very endearing way.

*"The patients hadn't gone home intending to die, but rather with the attitude of if only I have one year to live, how do I want to live it?* **Not** *dying was simply a side effect of living alive when loved fearlessly and without apology."*

If you are looking for a guide to help you "beat the odds" of immune disorders, abandonment issues, and chronic self-sabotage, this book is for you.

*"For the first time in my life, I wasn't running from my disease—I was running towards something greater: my wholeness."*

Loved it!

—**Julanne Dalke**, author of #1 Amazon Bestseller, *Your Eternal Identity, Practicing the Principles of a Spirit Supplied Life.* Contributing author of International best seller, *The Art of Connection, 365 Days of Gratitude and The Imaginist.* https://Julannedalke.com

As a gastroenterologist who has cared for countless patients over the decades, I know how deeply people search for clarity and hope when illness overwhelms. *Gut Instincts* offers both. It provides readers with a steady guide inward, offering tools and encouragement that make the path to healing feel possible again—a compassionate, practical companion for when nothing else seems to help.

—**Mark Reichelderfer**, MD & Professor of Medicine, University of Wisconsin-Madison

Jennifer Juniper writes with raw honesty and hard-won wisdom. Watching her live this transformation, and now seeing her share it so generously, reminded me why stories of real human courage matter most.

—**Amber Nolan**, screenwriter, director, producer

As a former national coach, I know firsthand the impact of the mind on physical health and performance. Gut Instincts is a remarkable piece of work—Jennifer brings together instinct, intuition, and deep wisdom to illuminate the mind-body connection and the healing power of thought. Her writing is insightful, uplifting, and an absolute joy to read.

—**Denise Holland**, Human Performance Consultant, speaker, author of *Play Freely*, and former national coach for Scotland Netball

Gut Instincts is for those who have ignored their gut, literally or figuratively, for years. It's never too late to come back to yourself. Follow Jen's lead. You will not be disappointed.

—**Kristina Neihouse**, author of the *Knowing When to Leave* trilogy

# GUT INSTINCTS

A Journey to Radical Healing,
Inner Knowing & Rewriting the Rules

## Jennifer Juniper

Goodyear, Arizona

# Dedication

I dedicate this book to my dad, who passed on the gift of writing and opened the door to so much more.

And to all the Crohn's and colitis sufferers out there who are—quite frankly—sick of this shit.

*Knocking at the door*
*It opens*
*I have been knocking from inside*
~Rumi

# Author's Note

This book is rooted in my experience with Crohn's disease, but it's about how trauma gets stored, and, if left unresolved, keeps us stuck. And it is written for anyone who's been dismissed, disbelieved, disorientated, or defined by the past.

Whether you have a body that is breaking down, a mind that won't quiet, emotions you can't escape, a spirit you feel disconnected from, a relationship repeating old patterns, work that isn't your passion, or a life that just doesn't feel like yours.

If you carried shame about what your body, mind, and/or spirit needs, how it behaves or what it reveals—this story is for you.

**Note to the reader:**
*This book explores difficult terrain—self-harm, suicide, and childhood abuse (emotional, physical, and sexual). These stories are shared in service of healing, but they may be activating. Please take care of yourself as you read.*

This book is an invitation to turn inward.
Scan the QR code below to access your gift:

*Inner Knowing Visualization*
—a short, guided experience to ground you and align your energy for the journey ahead.

## Claim Your Free Gift!

"At the center of your being, you have the answer;
you know who you are
and you know what you want."
~Lao Tzu

# Table of Contents

Endorsements ............................................................................................... 1
Dedication ..................................................................................................... 7
Author's Note ............................................................................................... 9
Before We Begin ........................................................................................ 15
Foreword by Jack Canfield ...................................................................... 17
Intro & Ignition .......................................................................................... 19

### Part One: Recognition
Uncover What's Lurking Behind Your Symptoms and Patterns
*Facing the truth: Go beyond surface problems to root causes
—it's the subconscious's way of telling a deeper story.*

**Chapter 1—Broken Horses:** The Art of Surrender .................................. 31
    *When the body breaks, so does the illusion of control.*

**Chapter 2—How Long (Has This Been Going On?)**
The Body Keeps Score ................................................................................ 39
    *Persistent patterns don't start the moment you notice them—
    they're the accumulation of years of stress, trauma, and
    unspoken pain.*

**Chapter 3—The First Cut Is the Deepest:** Wounds That Shape Us ...... 51
    *The wounds we don't address become the stories our bodies tell us.*

**Chapter 4—Like A Prayer:** Finding Spiritual Strength .......................... 59
    *The power of faith, intuition, and ethereal guidance in healing.*

**Chapter 5—Mother, Mother:** Carrying the Weight of
a Parent's Wounds ..................................................................................... 67
    *The weight of expectation, approval, and the longing for maternal love.*

**Chapter 6—Teenage Wasteland:** Self-Destruction as a Response to Pain .................................................................................................. 73
    *Rebellion, addiction, and the need to numb.*

**Chapter 7—Send Me an Angel:** The People Who Save Us and the Ones Who Almost Destroy Us .................................................. 81
    *Angels don't always have wings*

By the end of Part One, you'll see struggles as intel<br>
rather than problems to fix, and start recognizing the patterns<br>
that have been running beneath the surface.

Part Two: Reconnection<br>
The Art of Deep Listening<br>
Transformation begins when we move from opposition<br>
to collaboration with our inner intelligence.

**Chapter 8—Hell is for Children:** Breaking the Chain of Generational Trauma .................................................................................. 93
    *Approval equals love, performance establishes worth, rebellion and self-harm help you survive.*

**Chapter 9—Into the Mystic:** Awakening to Your True Nature ............ 101
    *Where self-discovery meets the spiritual, and we remember we are more than we thought.*

**Chapter 10—Another Brick In The Wall:** The Paradox of Self-Protection .............................................................................................. 111
    *What we build to keep pain out often keeps healing from getting in.*

**Chapter 11—Go Your Own Way:** The Power of Choice ...................... 121
    *True direction comes from turning down the volume on others' voices and tuning into your own.*

**Chapter 12—Breaking Point:** When Your Inner Wisdom Demands to be Heard .............................................................................. 131
    *When keeping it together falls apart there is beauty in the breakdown.*

**Chapter 13—Doctor!** The Limits of Denial ............................................. 139
    *What happens when the "experts" don't have the answers? Who do you trust then?*

**Chapter 14—I Need A Hero:** Some Battles Can't be Fought Alone ..........147
*When hope and desperation collide.*

**Chapter 15—Help!** The Fear of Knowing ...........................................................153
*When you're ready but they're not.*

By the end of Part Two, you'll shift from resistance to receptivity, learning to interpret your experiences as information not attacks.

### Part Three: Reclamation
Stepping Into Full Transformation & Freedom
*True liberation is not just about fixing what's not working
—it's about reclaiming your life.*

**Chapter 16—Don't Stop Believin':** The Power of Decision ........................... 163
*Healing starts with choosing to believe it. Others give opinions, but only you decide what's possible.*

**Chapter 17—Landslide:** The Collapse Before the Clarity ............................171
*When everything feels like it's falling apart, sometimes it's clearing the way or something new.*

**Chapter 18—You Learn:** Two Types of People ............................................. 181
*Some accept the prognosis. Others explore possibilities.*

**Chapter 19—Another One Bites the Dust:** The Cycle of False Hope ..... 189
*When the solution becomes a trap, it's time to find another way.*

**Chapter 20—Bullet With Butterfly Wings:** Breaking the Cycle ................197
*True freedom begins when you stop repeating the patterns that broke you.*

**Chapter 21—Start Me Up:** It's Not *What* You Eat, but *When* .......................203
*Those first baby steps create massive leaps down the road.*

**Chapter 22—I Want to Break Free:** The Power of Belief............................ 211
*Liberation from old identities*

**Chapter 23—Let's Get (Meta)Physical:** Getting to the Root ....................... 221
*Real healing happens when you stop treating the surface and start discovering the source.*

**Chapter 24—Digging in the Dirt:** What You Bury, Your Body Remembers ................................................................................................... 233
*Vulnerability, emotional healing, and the process of alchemizing past wounds.*

**Chapter 25—Changes:** Rewiring the Mind for Healing ....................... 243
*What you feed your mind is even more important than what you feed your body.*

**Chapter 26—Runnin' Down a Dream:** From Seeking Answers to Trusting Instincts ............................................................................................ 251
*Finding your way by following what resonates.*

**Chapter 27—The Sound of Silence:** Your Center in the Storm ................ 261
*The stillness you cultivate in calm becomes your anchor in chaos.*

**Chapter 28—Don't Give Up:** Rewriting the Rules .................................. 269
*When there's no way forward, you have to make one.*

**Chapter 29—This Woman's Work:** The Mind as Medicine ..................... 277
*Integration, complete ownership, and advocacy.*

**Chapter 30—Times Like These:** When Inner Knowing Becomes Unshakeable ............................................................................................... 287
*Sovereignty, self-trust, and stepping fully into your power.*

By the end of Part Three
you will recognize patterns and symptoms as messages, reconnect with your inner wisdom, and reclaim complete authority over your life.

**Epilogue—Best of You:** From Surviving to Thriving ................................ 295
*Trauma turned into a self-healing superpower*

**About the Author** ............................................................................................ 301

# Before We Begin...

**Dear Fellow Rebel,**

I see you.
    I believe you.
        I believe *in* you.
            And I'm rooting for you *all the way*.
                You are not alone.

Before you turn another page, I want you to know something:

You can do this.
I was once where you are, and I can help you get out.

Inside these pages, you'll find trauma wrapped in story, healing woven through memory, and truth spoken in a voice that's done apologizing.

Some chapters may stir you. Some may hold you.
Others may reflect what you've been feeling for a very long time.

My words are not meant to diagnose or instruct but to *mirror, unearth*, and *ignite*.

You are sovereign here.
Take what serves. Leave the rest.

## JENNIFER JUNIPER

    Pause.
        Cry.
            Skip.
                Rage.
                    Return.
                        You can't do this wrong.

Welcome to your journey through the body's love language, the mind's knowing, and the spirit's refusal to forget who you are. A journey as unique as you are.

It's about what the body remembers when the world refuses to listen.

    You've got this.
        And I've got you.

*Jen*

# Foreword

Every once in a while, a book comes along that doesn't just inspire you—it redefines what you thought was possible.

*Gut Instincts* is one of those books.

When I first encountered Jennifer Juniper's story, I was struck by the same quality I've seen in some of the most transformational leaders I've worked with: an unshakable decision to take full ownership of her healing, even when every external voice told her it couldn't be done. That decision—to stop outsourcing her power and start listening inward—is the foundation of the remarkable journey you're about to read.

As someone who has taught the principles of personal transformation for decades, I've always emphasized the power of decision, clarity, and responsibility. What Jennifer offers in these pages is that power, delivered from the raw terrain of lived experience.

It's a field guide written by someone who walked through fire and lives to light the way.

Jennifer's story is both deeply personal and universally resonant. She invites you into the intimate moments of her pain, her resistance, her breakthroughs—and most importantly, her return to self. Her voice is bold, poetic, irreverent, and full of heart.

She doesn't offer you a protocol. She provides you permission. Permission to listen. Permission to trust yourself.

Permission to believe that healing is not just possible, but yours to claim.

It moved me when I learned that one of my early audio programs played a pivotal role in Jennifer's healing journey. At the time, she had been addressing her illness solely through the physical body—doing everything she could to manage symptoms, chase treatments, and seek answers. What shifted in that moment was profound: she began to understand the role of the mind. The stories she was telling herself. The beliefs she was carrying. The energy of possibility. It changed everything. And that shift is one she now offers others, not as a concept, but as lived truth.

*Gut Instincts* isn't just a memoir. It's a reclamation. Of body. Of voice. Of truth.

If you've ever struggled with chronic illness, shame, confusion, or the quiet ache of not being seen, this book will speak to you in the language your body already knows. And if you're ready to stop chasing answers and start reclaiming your inner authority, you're holding exactly what you need.

Jennifer Juniper is the real deal. And this book has the power to change your life.

—**Jack Canfield**, Coauthor of the *Chicken Soup for the Soul®* series and *The Success Principles™: How to Get from Where You Are to Where You Want to Be*

# Intro & Ignition

*It's kind of fun to do the impossible.*
~Walt Disney

**How this book is different...**

There is a place in you where nothing is impossible.
Trust it.
I don't care what the experts told you, what other people say, or how many failed starts you've had. You have more influence over your health, your life, and your future than you've been led to believe.
I know because I've been where you are. Searching for answers, sifting for guidance I could trust, juggling advice and trying to make someone else's cookie-cutter system fit my unique shape—and still feeling stuck. Like something was missing.
When I stopped looking outside myself and turned my attention and efforts inward, I found a way through.
I wrote *Gut Instincts* to offer you that same path. A path to your inner wisdom and guidance. To the place that already knows exactly what you need and has the power to achieve it.
This book isn't here to give you another rigid plan. It's here to remind you that you already have everything you need to have whatever you want. You only need *discover* it

by getting to the root cause of your problems and removing the blocks in the way of your success.

A wise chiropractor that I know prepares patients for their first adjustment by saying, "Your body is a basement. It stores everything you're not able to deal with. Healing is the unpacking of those boxes. Be prepared to release and align on more levels than the physical."

I'm calling a sacred rebellion against surface-level models. We're going deeper, with tools that adapt to whatever the body/mind/spirit is flagging.

## What Does Healing Mean?

Healing is so much more than relief from symptoms. It's reclaiming your voice, your power, and your inner compass. Healing isn't just fixing what's broken. It's a return to wholeness, to the truth of who you are underneath the symptoms, stories, and survival patterns. It's remembering your natural state before fear, conditioning, and crisis took the wheel.

In this state of wholeness, you don't just feel better; you live differently. You choose differently. And you trust yourself in a way that makes every part of life more aligned and alive.

Healing is about getting to the root so it doesn't grow back. We're not just making your body behave, quieting your mind for a moment, or patching up your relationships until the next storm—we're restoring your relationship with *yourself*. Because when that's strong, everything else falls into place.

The relationship you have with yourself is the prototype for all the others. When you're good with you, your decisions get clearer, your energy feels lighter, and your life expands.

Healing is about living from the inside out—playing offense instead of defense, steering your life instead of merely reacting to what's coming at you. When you trust yourself at the deepest level, you stop chasing and start creating the life you want.

Healing is *not* linear. It's also not about pushing harder, following every rule, or proving yourself. It's about learning to hear, and *trust,* your own inner compass—even when the world tells you to hand it over.

Healing isn't about going back to how you used to be, but forward into more of who you really are. It's not a destination, rather a creative journey. It's more art than science, and that's where most people get it wrong. I did.

I spent years stumbling in the dark with Crohn's disease, doing everything right and getting sicker. Then came a glimmer. One note of truth that resonated through the noise. I followed it, and it grew into a chorus—one that sung me home to myself.

And it didn't end there.

I've used The Gut Instincts Healing Method™ ever since to navigate addiction, various existential crises, relationships, career changes, family of origin dynamics and most recently, menopause. These tools don't just get you through a crisis; they become a superpower to help you win every challenge.

Crohn's forced clarity. Louise Hay was right, I could heal my whole life. My disease *had* symptoms, but it also *was* a symptom of my entire ecosystem. That's why medicine alone failed. Most doctors only looked at the part of me presenting, carving it out and disregarding the rest—seeing the body as separate from the mind.

Getting incurably sick did what no accolade or achievement ever could—made me love myself. The healing process showed me that my value doesn't depend on producing or performing, and that's what ultimately set me free.

Today, Crohn's isn't even in my vocabulary, except to help someone. I'm a world traveler now, no longer chained to a toilet or even my own country.

I've eaten from street carts in Colombia without fear, biked fifty-six miles through the rolling hills of Wisconsin's farm country. I crossed the Vail Pass in a blizzard—in a *Honda*, parasailed over the Gulf of Mexico off a boat with no bathroom.

My amazing life used to feel impossible. I envied it in others. Now I give thanks for it every day.

This book is born from that transformation. A transformation that began by realizing that symptoms are the body's love language.

A nurse practitioner of integrative medicine put it like this: "The body is a communication device. It starts with a whisper, and it gets louder and louder until you hear it. It'll scream if it has to."

Symptoms are an invitation to start unpacking and a sign that you're ready. Ready to level up. You're here because you suspect there's something more—and you're right.

Let me be clear: this isn't a How-To book. It's a *Now-You* book.

Because the best anyone can do, and it's a beautiful thing, is to help activate your greatest healing power: the innate healing forces within.

> *The natural healing force within each of us*
> *is the greatest force in getting well.*
> ~Hippocrates

Right now, you might be giving that power away without even realizing it—to a doctor, a relationship, an influencer, a

## GUT INSTINCTS

fad, a supplement, a parent. But the truth? The things you try work or don't, according to your say-so.

That's what The Placebo Effect demonstrates: the power of belief. Seventy percent of study participants get better when given sugar pills because they were told it was medicine, and they *believed it*.

On the flip-side, The Nocebo Effect shows how belief in a doctor's warning about side effects can make your body create them.

Both are the power of belief at work.

It all starts with belief. Belief that everything can heal. Everything. Belief that your mind is powerful; your spirit, unlimited. Belief that life can be bigger, freer, and more loving and joyful than you've ever imagined.

Beliefs like that change the game. Belief, combined with decisive action, can rewrite your reality.

That saying, I'll believe it when I see it—it's actually the opposite. You'll *see it when you believe it*.

This book helps you leverage the power of belief and turn up the volume on your inner knowing.

By weaving your story alongside mine—I offer it for reference and recognition—you'll see what a reclamation journey looks like. You'll realize how childhood survival strategies shape adult patterns—patterns that can be cleansed.

Whatever made you sick, disconnected, unhappy, or stuck is the very thing that can set you free, returning you to vitality, clarity, harmony, and unity.

The world is full of people who've done this.

I sailed with a man who was told he'd never walk again after a catastrophic car accident. He not only came aboard easily, but had the most joyous and appreciative outlook on life.

I met a woman who reversed breast cancer in a month by micro-dosing apricot kernels after aligning her mind with story after story of others overcoming impossible odds and healing.

Jim Carrey, while broke and working as a janitor in L.A., drove to Mulholland Drive every night to visualize being a successful actor. He wrote himself a $10 million check for "acting services rendered" and dated it for 1995. By 1994, he'd landed *Dumb and Dumber*, *The Mask*, and *Ace Ventura*.

A friend confided over brunch her experience being hospitalized and diagnosed with ulcerative colitis. She refused surgery, went home and told the toxic partner and her violent son—she knew the stress was making her sick—to leave. She never had a symptom again.

Sara Blakely sold fax machines door-to-door, failed the LSAT twice, then cut the feet off pantyhose and turned the idea into Spanx. Starting with $5,000 in savings and zero fashion background, she became the youngest self-made female billionaire. "Mindset is the single most important thing you have. Work on it daily."

Mel Robbins struggled with crippling anxiety, unemployment, and drinking too much. She created the "5 Second Rule" to break her own cycle of self-sabotage and is now a bestselling author and speaker.

Then there's Joe Dispenza. He shattered six vertebrae after being hit by a truck when riding his bicycle. Surgeons told him he'd need complex surgery and would likely never walk again. Instead, he leaned on what he calls *the intelligence that made the body* to rebuild his spine mentally. He modeled his healed body internally until his external reality changed. His spine made a full recovery.

# GUT INSTINCTS

They're not superheroes. They're people just like you, with different backdrops and the same core truth: our mind is more powerful than our circumstances.

## How to Use This Book
I don't want you just to read this book and think, 'Wow, that was inspiring. Good for her.'

Inspiration without action is just a nice feeling you forget by Tuesday.

Here's how to actually *use* what's inside:

## Follow the Flow
The three phases—Recognition, Reconnection, Reclamation—build on each other. Skipping around is like trying to frost a cake before you've baked it.

## Do the Prompts
The questions and exercises are the bridge between *knowing* and *doing*. Write them down. Speak them out loud. Do them messy. Just do them.

## Don't Let Resistance Dissuade You
In my experience, if something feels uncomfortable it's because it's bumping up against an old pattern that needs to go.

*The obstacle is the way.*
~Zen saying

## Come Back Often
Your perspective will change. A chapter that's interesting now might be a lifeline six months from now.

## Why Now Matters

Every day you repeat the same patterns is another day you surrender your power—to symptoms, to old stories, to the belief that someone else holds the answers.

The longer you wait, the more those patterns dig in. And when they dig in, they don't just drain your energy; they shape your choices, your relationships, the way you see yourself.

But the moment you decide to step in, really step in, things start to shift. You begin to hear yourself more clearly. Your energy changes. You stop bracing for the next crisis and start creating something better.

This isn't about hustling for a quick fix. It's about reclaiming years of your life you don't want to lose to fear, fatigue, or someone else's definition of what's possible.

You can wait for the "perfect time," or you can start now.

And starting now is how you change everything.

## Your Healing Roadmap

This book is designed as a journey in three phases.

Think of it as moving from the outside in. From identifying what's running your life, to reconnecting with your true self, to reclaiming your full power.

**Phase 1 — Recognition:** Uncover what's behind your symptoms and patterns
- See beyond surface problems to root causes
- Spot the beliefs, behaviors, and stressors quietly draining you
- Name the patterns you've been living without realizing it

**Phase 2 — Reconnection:** Build trust in your own voice and wisdom
- Understand your body's love language
- Strengthen your relationship with your intuition
- Practice self-trust in small, doable ways

**Phase 3 — Reclamation:** Step fully into your authority and create your personal healing path
- Choose aligned actions with confidence
- See a prognosis as possibility, not certainty
- Live from your wholeness, not your wound

Inside each phase, we'll move through the five pillars of the **Gut Instincts Healing Method™**
1. *Feel* — body awareness, tuning in
2. *Face* — truth, trauma, old beliefs
3. *Filter* — intuitive discernment, boundaries
4. *Follow* — aligned action
5. *Free* — integration, release, identity shift

    Your path will be unique, but this structure will keep you oriented.
    What are you waiting for? Haven't you suffered enough?

Let's get started!

# JENNIFER JUNIPER

Scan the Code Below to View the Video for Intro and Ignition
Or go to: https://youtu.be/h31ofYUL7yl

Part One

# Recognition

## Uncover what's lurking behind your symptoms and patterns

*Go beyond surface problems to the root causes —it's the subconscious's way of telling a deeper story.*

## You Don't Have to Do This Alone!

As you work through this book, you might find yourself wanting to go deeper—or connect with others walking this path.

Explore one-on-one coaching and group programs at:
www.jenjuniper.com

# Chapter 1

# Broken Horses

**The Body Keeps Score**
When the body breaks, so does the illusion of control.

*Only broken horses know to run.*
*~Brandi Carlile*

My insides screamed and scraped like they were digesting razor blades dipped in Tabasco sauce. That should have been enough to get me out of the truck, up the ramp, and into the hospital doors right there, just on the other side of the curb—automatic, effortless doors swooshing open to welcome me.

The horseshoe driveway was built for ease and the quick pace of swooping in and dropping off those needing the most urgent of care. EMERGENCY blazed above, red hot and beckoning: *Bring me your broken, your hurting, your yearning to be free... of symptoms.*

But there was a sea between me and those doors—filled with shame, secrecy, and self-doubt. I had to protect that sea, so there was no easy drop-off for me. I got hung up on that horseshoe every time.

I was afraid something was seriously wrong with me, but I was more fearful of what they'd do to me to find out. I felt bad, and I felt bad about feeling bad. The pain doubled me over, coupled with the weight on my shoulders. At nineteen, the expectation of perfection had followed me out of childhood. I straddled and struggled with two ideas: taking responsibility for my health and my M.O. of self-protection.

One of the E's in *EMERGENCY* flickered, matching my nerves and mirroring my indecision. On and off. 'Are you in or out?'

"Come on," my boyfriend Josh soothed, patient as ever. "They're doctors. I'm sure they have something they can give you to make you feel better. Let's go in and talk to them." The lenses on his glasses were thick, set inside silver wire rims, making his eyes appear big and boyish.

My forehead rested against his dash in a puddle of sweat. Moans moistened the glove compartment. Food scraped and savaged its way through my intestines like it was shredding them apart.

*They'll want to do more than talk, and we both know it.* I held myself around the waist, pressing down, as if I could force my intestines into submission through sheer will. I took deep, controlled breaths. It worked sometimes.

I couldn't grasp his sense of security. I was all alone, locked inside an all-consuming pain. In a setting where it was their job to help the hurting, existing to hear the line, 'Something's wrong with me,' I still couldn't bring myself to say it. That was weird because I'd been sick a lot—from two to twenty-two—and I'd said it plenty of times. Maybe I'd also developed a pretty high tolerance.

Maybe it was too high.

Josh's easygoing nature was a big part of my initial attraction to him, and I counted on it when I wanted to be in control—which was often. In the heart monitor of our relationship, he was the straight line, and I the jumpy one, spiking above and below it in some chaotic pattern. I steadied myself against his steadiness, and he received frequent injections of excitement and exuberance from me.

Out of the corner of my eye, I saw people going in—limping, leaning on a loved one, holding a bandaged body part. I marveled at them like they were a different species. *How are they walking into the unknown like that?*

I barely talked about it with those close to me, much less strangers. It was my dirty little secret. And it was dirty.

Sickness puts you in a bubble, invisibly walled off from the normal world. But when it's your butt and bowels, that wall thickens. The vocabulary for the digestive system is embarrassing—gas, poop, diarrhea, rectum—it's gross and even more isolating. Especially for a young person, and especially for me.

We kept secrets in my family. We showed one face to the public and a very different face behind closed doors. Self-preservation was what was really going on. My family didn't look like other families. I'd felt something was wrong with me from a young age; my belly not working as it should was the icing on a multi-layered cake of deviations.

In addition to being violently, incessantly ill, I was filled with shame. Shame upon shame. This was the subfloor, covering a basement of shame—cobwebby, dark, dank.

I wished it were another part of my body breaking down—any other part. That would make it easier to talk about, at least. *Okay, maybe not my vagina.*

But I would have swapped with cancer.

I groaned, "Remember what Brenda told me they did to her?"

When my dad's girlfriend was my age with my symptoms, she had a colonoscopy. And when she woke up before it was over, the doctor dismissed her pleas to be put back under with a 'Hang in there, we're almost done.'

Judging by the storm clouds darkening her eyes, the trauma of it hadn't yet abated.

The doors gasped shut.

I wielded that story like a shield, rocking back and forth behind it and mentally counting the cramping in seconds. Partly as distraction and partly as self-diagnosis: How long did they last? Longer than the last time? Shorter? Hopefully shorter.

It was never shorter.

"That was a long time ago, Jen. I'm sure things have changed." Josh's tenderness was touching, and he displayed such patience, as if he were saying his well-worn line for the first time.

But we did this dance often, on the really bad days. And on really, really bad days, we sometimes did it twice. When pain hijacked our plans—its barbed-wire lasso tightening with every move—until I finally cried, 'Uncle,' and Josh would ask if I wanted to go to the emergency room. In quick response to my shallow breathing and reluctant nod, he'd make a detour to the nearest hospital, and those doors would swish open to welcome and woo me once again.

But I was frozen. Not physically—although that part would've been a challenge—my will stayed stuck in the gear, I Don't Need Anyone's Help and Wouldn't Know How to Ask Even If I Did. I was adamant, as always, making my case for this not being the right time. I had a paper due. A test to study for. Clients counting on me. We had dinner reservations. Friends awaiting our visit. The truck needed an oil change.

Anything but going in there and telling someone, "My poop comes out of me like a faucet on full blast."

If secrets and self-preservation were the bricks and mortar of my upbringing, then determination and fierce independence were the cornerstones. We sat there, I in my uncomfortable comfort zone, clinging to some shred of control—and if I'm honest, dignity—while looking out the window at those doors, representing a trust I couldn't muster.

I didn't want to talk to some strangers about my shit. Doctors overwhelmed me with all their needles, instruments, and hard-to-understand words, not to mention the ability to render one unconscious (or choose not to, and make you suffer).

The doors slapped close for the last time, dejected. From my bent-over angle, the fuzzy black fringe between them looked like eyebrows scrunched together in confusion.

I handled everything on my own. Everything. On my own. That was how I'd survived. My body wanted me to drop all that and turn myself in to the authorities? I couldn't do it. I didn't know how. I lacked whatever thought was needed to command my body.

I couldn't find the bridge.

---

**Core Theme / Emotional Wound:** *Control vs. vulnerability—* the fear of asking for help, resistance to surrender, shame around needing care.

**Old Survival Pattern:** *Hyper-self-reliance, masking pain* to avoid being "a burden" or seeming weak.

**Gut Instincts Healing Stage:** *Face.* Confronting the emotional armor that kept you "together"—but also isolated and unseen.

**Reflection:**
Sitting hunched in that truck, negotiating with pain and clinging to control, I was facing more than a medical crisis. I was standing at the door of a deeper healing, one that had

nothing to do with prescriptions or procedures. Looking back now, I see it clearly: I wasn't just resisting help from a hospital. I was resisting help, period.

Being raised on secrecy, silence, and survival, letting someone in meant knocking down a wall. What if everything I'd worked to hold together came undone? Maybe you've been there too—right on the threshold of help, but unable to take the step. Not because you didn't want to heal, but because you didn't feel safe enough to try. Explore your own barriers to healing—particularly around vulnerability, letting go of secrecy, and trusting support.

**Reader Reflection:**

1. **Threshold Moments:** What would it mean to let go of control and ask for help?
2. **The Mask of "Fine":** What secrets—physical, emotional, or otherwise—have you kept, in order to seem "fine"? (Fine stands for **F**eelings **I N**ever **E**xpress.)
3. **The Cost of Silence**: When have you ignored your own symptoms or needs because you didn't want to be "a problem"?

## Affirmations:

*I am safe in receiving help.*
*I am worthy of healing.*
*I do not have to hold everything alone.*
*I soften.*
*I open.*
*I receive.*

# GUT INSTINCTS

Scan the Code Below to View the Video for Chapter 1
Or go to: https://youtu.be/yQ0mQUvrnBs

# Chapter 2

# How Long *Has* This Been Going On

**The Body Keeps Score**
Persistent patterns don't start the moment you notice them
—they're the accumulation of years of
stress, trauma, and unspoken pain.

*The body keeps the score.*
~Bessel van der Kolk

In my junior year in high school life took turns coming together and unraveling in equally seismic ways. I was released early from a five-year stint in parochial school (*not* because of good behavior) and allowed to return to public school, where I never wanted to leave in the first place. The pause button on my relationship with my father toggled to play. And my body began breaking down.

A big year for a sixteen-year-old, and my belly absorbed the brunt of it. The chaos in my gut mirrored the chaos in my life.

I had very little power to wield around any of it. That's how it had always been. . .

Early one evening, late in the summer before seventh grade, my younger sister and I were racing to finish mowing the lawn before it got dark and the mosquitoes started their attack. Our mother crossed the lawn, not to tell us dinner was ready but rather, "I've decided you girls are going to Eastside."

The sun hung low behind her, casting an ominous glow over her pear-shaped silhouette—and the news.

Eastside Lutheran was the small school attached to the new church we'd started going to in Madison, fifteen miles away, instead of the church we'd gone to forever, just down the street.

Lisa and I stopped wrestling fresh grass clippings into collapsing Hefty bags to more fully voice our objections. We pleaded, then begged to stay at the school we knew, with all our friends and just a short bike ride from home.

What we wanted didn't matter.

"End of discussion," my mother adamantly uttered her well-worn phrase, even though no discussion ever happened. She made a statement, we argued, and she won. "School starts in two weeks," slammed like a gavel.

Mom's cutout was apocalyptic against the tangerine sky. With one sentence, she'd set fire to my life and severed the social network I tethered to—one of my few sources of stability in the tempest of my life. Friends I'd known and grown up with, from playing with dolls to hide and seek in the cemetery to learning to ride bikes and liking boys. From that safe harbor of the familiar, I sailed into uncharted waters.

I guess Mom didn't think I was weird enough already. Dissected from the rest of the class crafting a Father's Day card for my grandpa every year—salt in a gaping wound that I pretended didn't hurt—and forbidden by our church from joining Girl Scouts. I had to attend our church's version: Lutheran Girl Pioneers—no cool uniform with patches on the sash, no beret, no cookies.

I tried my best to sustain my friendships, but the commute to the church school meant I got home later, and our school breaks didn't line up. Two years later, I'm a freshman at an even further away Christian high school. I left in the morning in the dark, and when I returned home, it was dark.

The extra stretch and strain eventually snapped off my barely hanging-on hometown friendships completely. My new friends were scattered across small towns, far away, making meetups rare.

Lonely and feeling a little lost, I begged through the shower curtain for my sentencing to be overturned. Our conversations always happened while Mom was doing something else. Pleas rose with the steam, and my heart beat in wild desperation as I yelled. "I don't wanna learn about Jesus every day!!"

The shower curtain whipped open, metal hangers scraping as they flew down the rod. Naked, Mom sneered at me, revealing her silver-capped eye tooth—a sign that I was in big trouble. She jabbed a threatening finger into the damp air between us. "You better take that back!"

As if God would strike me dead for saying such a thing, pinning me to the vanity with a lightning bolt. Of course not. I didn't subscribe to all that fire and brimstone, always watching and vengeful, risk of eternal damnation crap. I believed in a good God; an all-knowing, all-loving, stay-by-your-side-in-case-you-need-help-with-anything, picking up the slack kind of God. But a vengeful God? *Nah.*

Even as a little girl, I'd reasoned it like this: I could get so mad at my sister that I'd wish she'd never been born, but send her to the flames of hell with the devil? She could never do anything to make me do that. And I wasn't even perfect. But I was supposed to believe a perfect, all-loving creator of the entire universe would?

It didn't make any sense. And whatever didn't add up in the equation, I subtracted out.

## JENNIFER JUNIPER

Learning about Jesus every day wasn't helping me, anyway. I'd gotten drunk at my very first football game. I started in the bleachers with my friends, cheering on my boyfriend—a freshman quarterback starting on the varsity team—when word came down the row that someone had brought a twelve-pack to the game. The invitation flipped an inner switch, and I let myself be pulled away from the game and under the bleachers.

Todd noticed my absence and, to my surprise, actually cared. I tried to fake it, but he'd had too many good plays, and I was a horrible liar. The following Friday night, outside the locker room before the game, I committed again to watching like a good girlfriend.

My butt locked into the bleachers until the lure of the party underneath became stronger than my promise. At home among the kids with speech impediments, one eye that wandered sideways, or a brother in jail, I looked up at the name-brand sneakers and perfectly curled hair of the kids in the stands. I knew I didn't belong up there.

By sophomore year, I was drinking every weekend and popping No-Doz out of my locker to get through the day. I finally wore my mother down, and she agreed to let me return to public school when I became a junior, if I still wanted to.

And I did. After school on my first day, I sat in the parking lot of Sun Prairie High School in the maroon Monte Carlo of my one remaining friend from my old life: Tony. I wanted to celebrate returning to where I never wanted to leave, but my head rested on the dash instead in a subservient pose to stomach cramps so intense they relegated my attention to only one thing: breathing. Arms tucked tightly across my middle, bracing me as wave after wave of pain broke on the shores of my stomach.

# GUT INSTINCTS

Tony and I had been friends since second grade. The only person safe enough to show my bad side to, inside the cocoon of our friendship—and his car. He passed me a joint. "Here," words straining against the smoke trying to escape, "maybe this'll help."

I moaned, turning and sliding on my sweaty forehead, cautiously unwinding an arm from a waistline getting chain-sawed in half. "I'll try anything." I reached for it not as a drug—surprising, given my fondness for altering my consciousness—but as medicine.

The stomachaches were getting worse and becoming more frequent. They were crampy like the flu, feverishly heating me and liquifying my insides as I hurried to the nearest toilet and explosively filled the bowl with the most godawful-smelling diarrhea.

*Shit never smells good, but mine smells toxic.* I didn't dare fart around anyone either—they were loud, long, and putrid. I'd either hold them in and hope no one heard the loud gurgling or use the bathroom pass to let them rip in solitude.

I exhaled out the window and into that after-school gap between the studious, aspiring, straight-A student me and the drinking, smoking, sneaking out of my bedroom window at night me. Pale smoke wafted out, filtering the view of the marching band practice where I should've been swooping and swirling my flag in rhythm to... my ears strained to hear through the haze... *Eye Of The Tiger.*

Pot relaxed my body and my mind, which worried about my body. Re-entering a social group after being out of the loop for four years wasn't as easy as I'd dreamed it would be. Or maybe I no longer belonged to the same group.

I'd left them as the stay-after-class-to-help-grade-papers-and-clap-chalkboard-erasers type and returned as the girl who carried a pack of Virginia Slims and kissed too many boys.

And now smoked pot.

Joining my friends again was like trying to merge onto the freeway on a tricycle. The intelligent, athletic kids were a tougher group to get into. I got good grades, but skipped school and found the princess superiority of Molly Ringwald's Claire too hard to maintain. The John Benders, however, were always recruiting. And they didn't do extracurriculars.

They barely did the curriculars.

But they had in free-flowing abundance things I desperately needed to relieve the pressure I was under: rebellion, acceptance—having fucked up and fragmented families was our common denominator, no need to pretend otherwise—and a whole variety of ways to sedate that developed right along with me. The viciousness of our world called for vices. We started forging a parent's signature to buy cigarettes. When that thrill wore off, we took up shoplifting, then clear booze (easy to replace with water), which blurred into making out with boys in the backseat—all tools in the toolboxes we had to carry because things were always breaking.

As I gained social stability, another surprise hit. My father reappeared.

Late one night, when my sister, mother, and I had just gotten home from one of my aunts' weddings and I was falling into bed pleasantly buzzed from all the champagne I'd snuck from half-finished glasses, the phone rang. *A call at two in the morning is never a good sign.* I strained to hear my mother's voice.

"Yes, this is she... Intensive Care... okay. We'll be right there."

# GUT INSTINCTS

A heaviness settled onto the side of my bed, making my body orient towards it. My room was dark, but where Mom sat was even darker.

The darkness sighed. "That was the hospital..."

I held my breath.

"It's your father," she whispered.

My body sank like she was sitting on my chest—or her words were. I didn't want to hear the rest. I would have kicked her off the bed, out of my room, and locked the door if I could have moved. But I was frozen and sticky hot all at the same time.

"He's been in a motorcycle accident. The doctors aren't sure he'll make it through the night. So, get up. Get dressed. We're going."

I was glad I was drunk. It softened the blow. Slowed down my mind so I could try to understand the bomb exploding inside of it.

Fervent prayers on the car ride shortened to a mantra as I burst through the hospital doors. *Live! Please. Live.* I pushed past the smell of sterility, desperation, and death clawing its way into my sinuses and gagging my sore and sandpapery throat. I squeezed helplessly into his room, greeted by grave faces and intensely operating machines.

In the middle of it all, my larger-than-life rock star dad looked frail with his head shaved, a plastic brace strapped to his torso, and an oxygen mask tied to his face. Seeing him lying there so eerily still triggered a deluge of tears. They distorted reality even more, like looking through a kaleidoscope.

The machines clicked and beeped, keeping him alive. Tubes ran like freeways, parallel and crisscrossed. My love swelled and contrasted with how little time I'd had with him—a sad, stark ratio clearing any lingering haze in my head. Our relationship was written in Morse code... dots of time together separated by dashes of distance—and just as hard to decipher.

The few memories I possessed conjured up and applied themselves like a balm. I carefully reached a shaking hand through the maze of tubes and touched his arm. "Dad? I'm here, Dad. I love you, Dad."

The machines answered. Click, beep.

"Please don't die," came out in snot and sobs. I tried focusing on the doctor's words, but my heart beat loud in my head.

"Rainy conditions. . . a curve. . . lost control. Coma. Next twenty-four hours. . . crucial."

I wanted to stay there for every minute of those hours, holding onto him and telling him how much I loved him. Praying. Pleading for him to open his eyelids and flash his smile that said everything was not only going to be alright, but awesome. A broad smile that wrinkled his nose, lit up his green eyes (just like mine), and showed the gap between his two front teeth—the same gap I had.

It was hard to hold onto hope in such a place, yet hope was all I had.

But the ICU is not for visiting. It is for last-ditch efforts on the dying, and a resurrection requires room.

We were out in the hall before the tears cried on his brace had dried.

I processed it the only way I knew how—through writing. Poetry specifically, in the margins of notebooks, in my journal at night, on the tender white part of my arm that never saw the sun. I took my poems to art class and practiced my calligraphy, transferring them onto poster board. After school, I'd gingerly tuck them under my arm, then tape them onto the walls of Dad's hospital room.

# GUT INSTINCTS

    Odes to a father I didn't really know but felt a deep connection with anyway. Proclaiming my love for him, summoning healing forces, heralding a relationship between us I'd stitched together from loose threads of memories kept safe in a corner of my heart. Anthems of encouragement to keep him fighting and confessions of my fear of losing him again.

    Hope and love, hope and love.

    School, then hospital. School, then hospital.

    Click. Beep. Click. Beep.

    Poems and prayers.

    That ICU room was a healing cocoon shut off from the rest of the world, where only family could enter. The four of us merged into the same lane again, where we had once been so many years ago.

---

**Core Theme / Emotional Wound:** *Disempowerment + identity disruption.* The trauma of having choices made for you, of losing connection to your voice and your people.

**Old Survival Pattern:** *Adapting to please others. Abandoning your own* needs, truth, and desires in order to maintain belonging, approval, or perceived safety.

**Gut Instincts Stage:** *Face* (with early threads of *Feel*)
Beginning to sense that your body is reacting to emotional dissonance—but not yet sure what it's asking for. It's the beginning of embodiment.

**Reflection:**
All the other people in that hospital scene—Mom, my sister Lisa, nurses, and doctors were in the wings. I felt alone as

the spotlight shone on Dad and me, highlighting the greatest ache.

My gut was carrying more than food. It was carrying the weight of everything I couldn't control. The forced silence. The emotional exile. The mask of perfection. My stomach was the first place that truth began to surface. I couldn't speak the words that hurt, so my body did. It started quietly, with cramps, stomachaches, and shameful symptoms, but the truth was always there, just under the surface. Looking back, I see now: my body wasn't the problem. It was the messenger.

Maybe your body has been holding things for you, too. Things you weren't allowed to express, question, or even feel. What if your symptoms aren't just problems to solve, but signals worth listening to?

**Reader Reflection:**

1. **Forced Silence:** When were you pulled out of alignment with your own identity, values, or community?
2. **The Body Speaks:** What did your body begin expressing when your voice couldn't?
3. **Losing and Reclaiming Voice:** Were there moments you felt like your truth didn't matter—or wasn't welcome?

## Affirmation:

*I reclaim my power by listening
to my body and honoring my truth.
I am free to rewrite my story.*

# GUT INSTINCTS

Scan the Code Below to View the Video for Chapter 2:
Or go to: https://youtu.be/cQ58fZgYnn0

## Chapter 3

# The First Cut Is the Deepest

### Wounds That Shape Us
The wounds we don't address become the stories our bodies tell.

*The wound is the place where the Light enters you.*
~Rumi

When you're little, the world is little and your parents loom large within it. At the center of my world was Daddy, especially on the nights my mom worked as a checker at the grocery store. He'd put my baby sister to bed, but I stayed up because I was two years older.

Those nights in the living room belonged to our daddy/daughter duets, with my dad on the sofa, softly strumming and me, twirling around and giggling to the melody until I got dizzy. I'd wobble to the coffee table to steady myself, then clap for more as soon as the room stood still. Daddy's long arms and legs sticking out from behind his guitar looked like the Itsy-Bitsy Spider.

Our dancing, singing, strumming, and laughing flowed as the clock ticked closer to the store's closing and my mom's return home. At the first flash of her headlights, the neck of the guitar would spin up and over my daddy's face while I made a run for my bed. He was close behind, scooping me up and tucking me in, both of us giggling.

"Shhhh," he'd put his finger to his lips while the other hand closed the door and I squeezed my eyes shut, feet still warm from whirling around on the carpet.

[It's the sensations I remember most: the specialness of our secret time together, the safety of his presence, the warmth of his love matching the warmth of my feet. Details were added later, when I was older and Dad told me the story.

But this next scene is etched so clearly that I need no one's help. The memory of it is so visceral, it has the power to slingshot me back to being four years old, covered in the hot skin pricks of apocalyptic dread.]

Blood rivered down Daddy's knuckles. Their fights weren't usually violent, and it wasn't what scared me most; the guitar slung across his back said he was leaving leaving. Was he telling us where he was going? I couldn't hear over the wailing that my mother, my koala bear of a little sister on her hip, and I were doing.

All I could do was watch helplessly as the person I loved the most and felt the most loved *by* took big steps across the living room, darkened into a silhouette against the large picture window, turned the doorknob and walked out of our lives.

I felt my whole world implode. I panicked as the four-year-old equivalent of, 'We are so fucked' coursed through my mind.

A heavy curtain fell on my life that day, the end of an act. Childhood was over. The notch where he'd punched their bedroom door greeted me whenever I came out of mine. Looming high above me, it looked like an open mouth, so I'd ask, *"Why did you leave, Daddy? Why?"*

## GUT INSTINCTS

Mornings, I looked at it hopefully telling myself, *Maybe today you'll come back.* Then the next day, *Today?* I'd try to soothe myself after brushing my teeth on the way to bed, *Maybe tomorrow.* As I grew closer to that hole, my questions grew, too. *Where are you? Why didn't you take me with?*

Time moved on, but I didn't.

That hole in the door marked a hole in my life that I fell through, like Alice in Wonderland. Our family rebranded as Debbie and The Girls, but I couldn't adjust. I found the Dad-shaped void in our family unbearable. Nothing could fill it.

No matter how many people were around or how great a thing was happening, it always felt like something was missing.

***

Those critical twenty-four hours of Dad in the ICU turned into days. I treaded lightly around this latest appearance of him, the steadiest his presence had been since he'd left, and found myself wondering where he'd been all those years. I totally got why he didn't want to be married to my mother, but not why he didn't want to be my father. Two deep wonderings swirled within me: how hard he tried to see me and how easy my mother made it.

But I wasn't asking either for fear he'd run off again. Or fly away like a butterfly I failed to get my net entirely over.

That's what happened the last time he came around. I was about twelve when our family reunited at a pizza place. My dad was just as tall as I'd remembered, with the same big smile under his big, black mustache and a playfulness that lifted all our moods.

I don't remember much of what was said. Shakey's Pizza Parlor had windows where you could see your pizza being made, and that's where my sister and I perched, watching spinning discs of dough get airborne and glancing at our parents talking back at the table.

That's how secure I felt in the reimagining of my family. Dad was back with the fun, Mom was laughing, everyone was happy, and everything would be okay from now on.

We were a family again.

Outside in the parking lot, we made plans for weekend visits after church on Sunday, I bounced and giggled with excitement and anticipation. After about a month my sister decided she didn't want to go, so it was just me and Dad—a duet once again.

Then it was every other Sunday.

Then, it was no Sunday at all.

Dad faded back out of my life the same way he'd faded in, with little explanation and zero space to process the emotional fallout—like so many things. I'd decided to handle it differently this time by telling myself it didn't matter, that I didn't need him. Sitting by his hospital bed, I felt like a kid again. My Dad dream locked and loaded, hoping upon hope that this would be the time it turned into reality that lasted.

Days passed and details of the accident filled in. Taking a turn too fast in the rain had thrown him from his motorcycle into a signpost; an impact so hard it bent the post and broke his back. He would live, but in a wheelchair, paralyzed from the waist down.

And then he was paralyzed from the hips down.

A few days later I entered the door of his hospital room and found him hoisted up on his hands, swinging his hips side to side. The big smile was back, along with 'look what I can do' excitement sparking in his eyes, all against the backdrop of a doctor looking bewildered.

I wasn't.

I was a big believer in miracles and knew they often occurred in precisely these kinds of circumstances. 'In God, all things are possible.' 'The peace that passeth all understanding.' The hymn *How Great Thou Art*. They weren't just words on a Sunday morning. They were invocations of faith to stabilize me when life got crazy, evocations of something ancient and authentic inside me.

Faith seemed like a deposit one made, then withdrew when times got tough.

So much love filled Dad's hospital room; piped in from the outside, too. Cards, balloons, and flowers surrounded us all, their warm wishes contrasting the cold metal of the machines and splashing color across the sterile white room. Even my mother, who'd only expressed hatred for the man; wouldn't even talk about him whenever I asked—which was often—except to say he'd probably gone to California to chase his dream of being a musician (*leaving me behind in a nightmare*) was now buying him hi-tops and smiling adoringly as she laced them onto his feet.

Gaining that extra six inches of movement didn't mean my dad could walk, but he could move around a lot easier, transferring in and out of his wheelchair independently. In gaining those inches, he'd gained freedom.

We left the ICU with fanfare and celebration. A regular room meant longer visiting hours and more people from Dad's vast social circle. Like coworkers from the newspaper where he worked as a music journalist, his girlfriend, members from the local and national bands he reviewed, promoted, and supported, his other girlfriend.

When my mom met the first one, I thought she'd rip those hi-tops right off his feet and whip them across the room. Eventually, both girlfriends visited at the same time. A snarl erupted, one stormed out, then the other, taking him from three female adorers to none—except for me. There was nothing my dad could do to alter my opinion of him. Most of his visitors didn't even know he had kids, a minor detail I brushed off.

"I swear, Jennifer, you have him on such a pedestal!" My mother accused. She never came into the hospital again, providing only transportation.

Her admonition did nothing to temper my gushing about him. About the strides he'd made, how funny he was, all the cool people he knew, how cool *he* was. Every day he improved, and the visits became more entertaining. I never knew which band or venue owner might be there to greet and meet. It felt more like a party. Dad's bed was his stage, his visitors his captive audience. Nurses fawned over him. Doctors loved him. Everyone loved him.

On one car ride home, I excitedly told Mom about an a cappella Canadian band called The Nylons visiting and singing to my dad, as well as signing autographs for the staff.

She clicked her tongue. "I think you're so desperate for a father, you'd have taken anything."

I ignored the sting of her words and the possibility of their truth, clung to the version I needed Dad to be, and tucked into the realization that tragedy and miracles had partnered up once before…

---

**Core Theme / Emotional Wound:** *Abandonment and loss of safety.* The sudden disappearance of trusted love creates a deep imprint in the body—a blueprint of grief, distrust, and unmet longing.

# GUT INSTINCTS

**Old Survival Pattern:** *Seeking external rescue* while internalizing the belief that love always disappears. *Learning to mistrust* joy, connection, and good things for fear they will vanish without warning.

**Gut Instincts Healing Stage:** *Feel.* Your body becomes the first container for grief—and the first receiver of spiritual reassurance, even before words or logic were available. Something inside you is still alive, still listening, even when the world outside goes silent.

**Reflection:**
At four years old, I didn't have the words for abandonment or trauma. I only had a body. And it remembered everything. It remembered the moment the music stopped, the door slammed, and the love I trusted disappeared.

This chapter marks the first emotional rupture: the sudden, visceral loss of my father, and with it, the loss of childhood innocence, belonging, and safety. My first existential crisis as the ground beneath me gave way to quicksand. My body began carrying the grief, the confusion, the unmet longing.

Maybe your body remembers, too. Perhaps it's been holding your unsaid truths, un-cried tears, and unmet needs all these years. Let's pause and listen.

The word a cappella means 'in the manner of the chapel.' This style originally referred to singing without accompaniment. Voices rising together, no instruments, *just soul and resonance in pure form*. Like the sound is sacred because it's stripped down.

Just like healing. Just like truth.

Tragedy invites us into our own a cappella work—no flashy tools, just raw you, aligned and vibrating in your own chapel of clarity.

Dad's was the first hospital-based miracle I'd witnessed, but it wouldn't be the last.

**Reader Reflection:**

1. **Listening to Early Signals.** Reflect on your earliest memories of feeling emotionally overwhelmed. Where did you feel it in your body?
2. **Living With Silent Pain.** Were you the child who cried easily, got stomach aches, or held it all in? What were you trying to digest that no one saw?
3. **Learning to Trust the Body's Voice.** Today, where in your body do you feel tension, tightness, or discomfort most often? If that body part could speak, what would it say?

## Affirmation:

*I can be free of the burden of unmet needs
and expectations from the past.
The love I seek is already within me.*

Scan the Code Below to View the Video for Chapter 3:
Or go to: http://y2u.be/1hTsD332hNs

# Chapter 4

# Like A Prayer

### Finding Spiritual Strength
The power of faith, intuition, and ethereal guidance in healing

*Faith is taking the first step
even when you don't see the whole staircase.*
~Martin Luther King Jr.

My first whole snippet of memory after my dad left is a random Polaroid—loose, without a photo album for context. He called for the first time, at least the first time I knew about. I was around eight years old, my childlike innocence still intact. I believed in Santa, wasn't sure if a watermelon would really grow in my belly if I swallowed a seed, and trusted everything the adults in my life told me.

"It's your father," Mom said matter-of-factly while handing me the phone, as if four years hadn't gone by without him. Four years of her introducing us as 'This is Lisa; she's *my* daughter. And this is Jennifer; she's her father's daughter.'

One glance and you could see she was right. My sister clung to her, comfortably nestled inside that designation, with eyes the same watery shade of blue as Mom's. I stood a little apart, with my green eyes and my mental casting about. *Then where is he? Where is my daddy so I can be his girl?*

## JENNIFER JUNIPER

Dad called to say he was diabetic and what the warning signs were because it's hereditary. "Tell someone if you get really thirsty or tired, okay?" His voice was deep and concerned, the timbre of which made something bloom inside me.

*Daddy does love me! He does!* His voice was in my ear again. He was in my life again, the tether between us tightening like it used to be.

"My blood sugar count was so high, the doctor said he was surprised I didn't melt in the shower!" His serious voice turned to a snicker. Picturing him melting down the drain made me giggle, which made him laugh, and then I laughed harder.

All I cared about, all I wanted, was to have Daddy back in my life. He said he would come to visit me "Tomorrow." Igniting a hope that nothing could put out.

Tomorrow was my new favorite day. Better than Christmas. Better than my birthday. Better than all my eight birthdays and eight Christmases and every Easter basket and every coin tucked under my pillow by the Tooth Fairy combined.

As soon as I got home from school, I tucked my super excited self into the chair in front of our big living room window—the same one he'd walked past when he walked out the door on the worst day of my life—and waited for him. The clock ticked 'any minute now, any minute now' and my imagination ran wild with what he would look like and what we would do, how it would feel to be in his arms again.

My eyes followed each car that turned down our street, wondering if it was his.

*Is this one him?* ... I squinted to see through the windshield.
Maybe the next one.
*This one?*
*Next one.*

# GUT INSTINCTS

*Next one? . . .*

I clung to his words as I waited. *He said he'd come.*

Pans clanked in the kitchen. I smelled the first hints of Mom cooking dinner. I gulped down my food and kept my eyes locked on the door. *Any minute now. He's going to walk in any minute now.* I even ate all my vegetables. Usually, I complained until Mom said I just had to eat as many as I was old, but even Brussels sprouts tasted good on my favorite day.

Mom tried telling me she wasn't sure if he was coming.

"Why would he say it then?" I didn't wait for her answer. I zipped right back to my perch and waited.

Waited and prayed.

Not the memorized *Now I Lay Me Down to Sleep* hanging embroidered above my headboard, performed nightly on my knees with hands clasped and without thinking—a more specific, simple one, beating in me like a drum.

*PleaseGodPleaseGodPleaseGodPleaseGodPleaseGod.*

My chest felt heavier and heavier. It felt like our kitty Sophie was sitting on it. As darkness crept in, I felt my heart breaking all over again, like a scab I'd picked and made bleed. I was lying in the chair now, my tears rolling out the side and wetting the arm. I pleaded as I sobbed, *Please come, Daddy. Please.*

In the sky, thick clouds started to form—matching my mood—and the falling rain created a waterscape on the window, mirroring the one on both my cheeks. I looked down at the grass and watched the wind move it back and forth, the raindrops making the clovers bend and then bounce back up. It rained harder, parting the grass and twisting the clovers into shapes.

Blinking my tears away, I squinted and tried to focus. I saw a nose first, and then an eye. I straightened from my slumping over the arm of the chair to get a better view. *Is that a face?* A beard came into focus, answering 'yes!' I leaned in farther, my forehead hitting, then resting on the cold glass to watch for more.

The scene became more defined with the little green face smoking a little pipe. A top hat completed the character, erasing all doubt. The leprechaun in the grass began dancing a jig. I giggled at this real-life Lucky Charms commercial happening before me, and *for* me.

My tears suddenly stopped. I felt all toasty inside, like in the warming house at the ice-skating pond in the park. When I got so cold trying to imitate Dorothy Hamill in the Olympics that my face hurt and I could no longer feel my toes, I'd clomp my blades up the wooden ramp, opening the door to a blast of warmth and nice old ladies handing me hot cocoa with mini marshmallows on top and calling me *Dear*.

I'd slip off my mittens, wrap my stiff hands around the foam cup, and tip the already melting marshmallows to my lips. The wood stove warmed me from the outside, and the hot chocolate heated my insides.

Daddy's car still hadn't pulled up. He hadn't burst through the door, scooped me up in his arms, and swung me around, calling me his princess and promising never to leave again. But inside it felt like it, plus all my other favorite things: Christmas, trick-or-treating, birthdays, dance recitals, sliding into clean sheets fresh off the line, warm, fluffy towels right out of the dryer.

*Something* had heard me and answered in a way I could understand. I felt loved. Safe. As if I were lying in the lap of God, not in a chair.

Who else could make the grass come alive and create a hot chocolate in the warming house scene without any hot chocolate or warming house? (It wasn't even winter!) The One who talked through burning bushes in the desert would be my first guess. Bible stories from Sunday School enthralled me: Jesus telling a crippled man to get up and walk, shepherds following a star across the desert, Jonah rescued from a whale.

What did Jonah have that I didn't have? I was trapped, too! That chair was my whale. My cries directed at the same God. If Jesus could make mud and help a blind man see, then surely he could handle bringing Daddy back to me. It seemed like a much easier task in my mind.

I'd happily drunk the Kool-Aid during the two weeks of summer that were Vacation Bible School, but I'd spit out the parts about God sending a flood or damning His creations to eternal burning hell. I couldn't believe in that kind of God. That kind of God was no good to me. I needed a fuzzy, soft teddy bear sort of God to cling to when I got scared—a holding hands and skipping to school kind of God.

In Sunday School, when the teacher told us the story of Jesus dying for our sins, I pictured it like a game of Kick the Can. We could all come out of hiding. We'd been set free. My hand shot up in excitement. "So, we're good, right?? Everyone goes to Heaven!" The excitement and relief were a heady mix.

"That's not exactly how it works. . ." Her voice trailed off as she handed out the popsicle sticks and glue to make crosses.

But something told me that had to be how it worked. If Jesus and His crown of thorns nailed to the cross weren't enough to save me, then what did she expect me to do—one better?

I thought of Grandpa, the main source of love and joy in the family. He only went to church on Christmas and Easter when Grandma made him, but he fished all the other Sunday mornings. *Would that be enough to save him?*

I told no one about my scene in the grass, afraid they'd say to me it wasn't real. Couldn't risk it. It was too valuable.

I couldn't afford to have yet another loving presence taken away from me. It would be mine and God's secret, tucked into my pocket for the next rainy day.

Salve spread on a wound doesn't make it go away instantly. My dad didn't magically appear either, but I felt better about it somehow—understood, deeply loved, and attended to anyway.

A firm foundation slid in beneath me. Compared to the mist of a mother and the fragmented appearances of my father, it seemed much more solid.

---

**Theme / Emotional Wound:** *Emotional abandonment.* Longing to be chosen, held—the medicine begins to arrive: an internal knowing that we're not alone. The *inner scaffolding starts* to form.

**Old Survival Pattern:** *Hiding intuitive, spiritual, or inner-truth experiences* to stay safe from judgment, ridicule, or abandonment. Learning to distrust the body's more profound wisdom in exchange for external approval and belonging.

**Gut Instincts Stage:** *Feel.* A profound moment of connection arises—not with people, but with something larger, loving, and real. This is intuitive knowing *before* language or logic.

**Reflection:**
That night, I waited for love to walk through the door. It didn't. But something else did—something soft, sacred, steady.

I didn't know the word "intuition" yet. I didn't call it Spirit. But I felt it plant the seed of unshakable love inside me. Looking back, I see God stepping in as the provider of unconditional love—the representation of a presence that would never leave me.

Maybe you've waited too—for someone to come back, for pain to be seen, for the ache inside to be held. Maybe, like me, what you need isn't always a person. Maybe what you need is already inside you, waiting to be felt. Even amidst deep loss, we're already rewiring for truth—and every time you listen to that quiet knowing, you lay another brick in your foundation.

## Reader Reflections:

1. **Longing for Love:** What's a moment from childhood when you longed for love that never came the way you hoped?
2. **Glimpses of the Unseen:** When have you felt something unseen step in and hold you, even if just for a breath?
3. **Hiding Inner Knowing:** Have you ever dismissed or hidden a spiritual or intuitive experience because you feared it wouldn't be believed?

## Affirmation:

*I am never truly alone;*
*love and comfort are within me, always.*

## JENNIFER JUNIPER

Scan the Code Below to View the Video for Chapter 4:
Or go to: https://youtu.be/oBkVpb5jUJU

# Chapter 5

# Mother, Mother

**Carrying the Weight of a Parent's Wounds**
The weight of expectation, approval,
and the longing for maternal love.

*I am whole, even when I feel misunderstood.
My worth is already established.*

If from my father's mouth broken promises fell, from my mother's came the familiar refrain, 'Come talk to me while I get ready for work." I trailed behind her, trying to get her to turn around. To give me her full attention, maybe even lift me into her arms and say, "I'm listening. Tell me everything."

But that was Fantasy Mom. Real Mom, fueled by the never-empty coffee pot on the kitchen counter, was always moving fast on her way to something, so that she could be on her way to something else.

I'd start cross-legged in the center of the bed, raving or ranting about my day, then relax into her pillows, releasing the scent of her—Chanel No.5. She'd slide her uniform out of the dry-cleaning bag with its familiar crinkle.

First came the bulletproof vest that squashed her chest and made her look like a man. Two belts, a regular one to hold up her pants and then a big, heavy one to hold the handcuffs, the club, a jangling keyring with keys I tried to count but there were way too many, extra bullets lined up like little soldiers, and a gun in the holster. I sort of checked them off mindlessly and continued the report of my day—a gauge of how much time I had left with her.

Was it habit or comfort? I didn't know, but it was part of the routine. I did it without thinking or flinching, and I did it every time. She worked two jobs, plus overtime—a cop in all of them. 'my mom, the cop,' was more like 'the cop, my mom.'

There was never enough time to process everything I needed to. I complained she never really listened to me, and she complained I talked too much.

I don't know how old I was when my sister and I began being left alone, but I was too young to get the Kraft Macaroni and Cheese right. Lisa would spoon up then pour the neon orange liquid and tease me with the Chunky Soup jingle, "It's the soup that eats like a meal!"

When mom was home, she often slept. Her bedroom door closed, my sister and I whispering and tiptoeing around, trying not to wake her. Because if we did, the sound of her turning the doorknob was a squeaky omen of the wrath unleashed on us for interrupting the little sleep she got. Her form would fill the doorway, lips parting into that sneer that revealed the silver-capped tooth—a gleaming fang.

First came the screaming, then the spankings (mostly me because, being older, I should know better), then our tears and promises to be better. To *behave*. But no matter how hard we tried, it was impossible. We were too young to be kept under wraps for too long. Our play eventually got rambunctious; a cupboard door would accidentally get closed too loudly, or we'd start fighting. And the ominous squeak of that doorknob would sound its warning shot.

# GUT INSTINCTS

As I grew older, I gradually became accustomed to the early onset independence and her strict discipline, but I couldn't get used to her disappointment. I kept trying, harder and harder, to make her proud of me.

I handed her my report card the second I got in the car. Maybe this time, I'd made her proud.

"What's this?" She pointed at the tiny dash, a deduction next to my **A**. "What did you miss?"

I felt my stomach drop. No praise, just disappointment.

I was unraveling right along with the run in my nylons that I was trying to hide under my skirt. The kids around me all seemed so happy and supported. Life was serious and hung heavy on me, even at the age of twelve. Having only one parent put me in the minority at a public school, but at a *Christian* school, it put me in a class all by myself.

In extracurriculars, I could blend in—same uniforms, working as a team, playing the same song in band. But when practice or rehearsal ended, they all walked home or carpooled, and I sat on the yellow curb waiting for my mom to come.

And waited.

And waited. I memorized the cracks in the pavement, tracing them with my shoe, waiting. First, the kids left. Then, the teachers. Then, the janitor. Eventually, I'd go into the church office and ask to use the phone to call home, but there was never an answer.

When I was sick, that's when I got the mom I wanted. Fantasy Mom. The world stopped if I wasn't feeling well, and all the places and things to rush off to disappeared, like magic.

I got ear infections, *a lot*. Even with tubes in my ears from toddler age, the ear infections continued to plague me. At five years old, they took out my tonsils, but the ear infections continued. I have countless memories of a hot water bottle being my pillow, and pressing my bad ear (I counted myself lucky if it was only one ear) against it for soothing relief as the towel wrapped around it absorbed my tears.

I'd close my eyes, bracing myself against the shock of the icy cold drops that sent the world underwater as they crackled loudly, bubbling and slithering their way through my ear canal. It felt them coming into my eyes, drowning me.

Mom would wrap around me, cuddling me from behind, stroking my hair, and humming to comfort me. I turned the throbbing in my ear into drumming, grasping for harmony within our rhythm and waiting for the deep, hot pain to stop. The scene is crystal clear, a timestamp of my toddler to pre-teen years.

A bottle of bubble-gum-tasting medicine lived in our fridge like a condiment: ketchup, mustard, and pink penicillin. Nothing helped, at least not for long.

*What is so wrong with me that I can't be fixed?*

---

**Theme / Emotional Wound:** *Inconsistent love + conditional safety = internalized unworthiness.* I'm only worthy of softness when I'm suffering.

**Old Survival Pattern:** *Believing love must be earned* through self-erasure—working harder, shrinking smaller, tying worth to performance or pain. Survival meant being useful, good, or broken enough to deserve care, while abandoning the parts of yourself that were messy, loud, or simply human.

**Gut Instincts Stage:** *Face*—not just the pain, but the pattern. The early conditioning. The reality that love was inconsistent and therefore unpredictable. The body is holding grief, vigilance, and confusion.

**Reflection:**
Sometimes, the deepest wounds aren't from what was done to us, but from what was withheld. When love was only offered on the condition of suffering, silence, or performance, it taught our nervous system that we had to earn care. That collapse or compliance might finally make us worthy.

Did you also learn your worth was determined by what you could endure? Perhaps you learned to become smaller, quieter, or sicker to deserve tenderness.

If so, you are not alone. And you are not broken beyond repair.

There is a different way to live. You don't have to suffer to be worthy of softness.

**Reader Reflection:**

1. **Conditional Care:** What early messages did you receive about when it was okay to need care? Did care feel freely given—or was it something you had to "earn" through being good, quiet, or sick? Was love in your home unconditional?
2. **Tying Worth to Performance:** In what ways have you learned to over-function, overachieve, or minimize your needs in order to feel safe, accepted, or loved?
3. **Untangling Love and Suffering:** Where in your life today do you still feel pulled to "prove" your pain to receive tenderness? What might shift if you allowed care without collapse?

## Affirmation:

*I am worthy of comfort without crisis.*
*I no longer confuse suffering with love.*

JENNIFER JUNIPER

Scan the Code Below to View the Video for Chapter 5:
Or go to: https://youtu.be/1j1CUKBeVwQ

## Chapter 6

# Teenage Wasteland

**Self-Destruction as a Response to Pain**
Rebellion, addiction, and the need to numb.

*In the middle of difficulty lies opportunity.*
*~Albert Einstein*

Between sixteen and moving out at seventeen, life was like a dam constantly springing leaks. I rattled through my toolbox often, scrambling through an arsenal of corks to plug the holes.

Up until my sixteenth Christmas, I thought I was the oldest. But that Christmas Day, at my grandparents' house, a revelation rocked my world once again. From the kitchen, I heard an argument brewing between my mom and her sister, Aunt Cathy. Voices rose to a crescendo, and tension charged the air like an approaching storm.

Months earlier, I'd answered a pounding on our kitchen door to find my ten-year-old cousin, Troy, clinging to our porch railing, his face deep red and flushed with tears. A large man followed, tried to pry him away, but Troy held fast, like a wild animal caught in a trap. I hadn't seen him in years. He'd quietly slipped from our lives, supposedly to go live with his dad. But later I learned he'd been in a foster home and was running away from abuse.

At Christmas, my mother offered to intervene, using her influence as a police officer and her position as the eldest in the family. But Cathy wasn't having it. The argument swelled, tension throbbed in my stomach as I braced myself. Cathy's voice exploded like a gunshot: "If you want a boy to save, go find Mark!"

Silence blanketed the house. Not a single fork tinged a plate, suspended in the weight of the secret my aunt uncorked. My mom was the oldest of ten—silence was unnatural.

"Girls, get your coats," she commanded, walking past us without looking back. She drove home in silence, the car thick with secrets. As soon as we got inside, she left again with a terse, "I'll be back."

In the stunned quiet, I dialed the one person who got me—my aunt Shelly. She reluctantly explained, "Your mom and dad had a baby before you. A boy. His name is Mark. That's all I know."

The shock gripped me, pulling at my sense of family and my place in it. My parents were young when they had me at nineteen, and I was stunned to hear that they'd had one when they were even younger. Hours later, Mom returned, clanging pots and pans in the kitchen as if nothing had happened.

"We have a brother?" I asked, steeling myself.

She stopped slicing mid-potato, her back remained turned. "If you love me, you'll never ask me about it again."

I swallowed my questions like poison, letting them settle into my stomach. If silence was the price of her love, I would pay it. But something shifted in me that night. A crack formed where trust had been.

The chasm between Mom and me deepened. I circumvented her 'You're just asking for it, dressed like that' by stuffing black leather pants and a lace top into my backpack and changing in the bathroom at school. Instead of arguing for the same curfew as my friends, I snuck out my bed room window.

The bright spot in my dark sky was Dad's accident, bringing a resurgence in our relationship. Weekend visits resumed. At Dad's, I had freedom—just needed to keep him in the loop. 'You don't need a father. But I can be your friend,' he said.

I didn't say it, but I thought I needed a father more than anything. I smiled like it was a gift instead of a wound. Anything was more than nothing. I didn't ask him about Mark, afraid of straining our fragile relationship. I figured I'd ask later, when we were more solid. I could wait.

We had time.

Our weekends together were a whirlwind of entertainment. Dad's wheelchair didn't stop him from taking me to concerts, where he always knew the sound guy or someone in the band. My sister and I watched the first of The Nylons' two-night run in our seats with the audience and the second, side stage, tucked between maroon velvet curtains that we were careful not to move when we danced.

I merged into his rockstar world of cool friends, countless bands, and smoking hash under a glass with Rastafarians while reggae wafted from the turntable. A mix called "Around the World" sent me into orbit. I snuck away to get grounded again on the bathroom floor, leaning against the wall and waited for the nausea and terror to pass. I didn't call for my dad, and he didn't check on me. I handled it alone. That's what I was learning from my barely-there parents.

On one of these weekends, a friend brought over opium. "This is serious stuff," Dad warned, uncharacteristically parental. Up until then, his big dad move had been, 'I'm not selling my daughter weed. Here, just take it.'

I watched my insecurities float away in a cloud of opium smoke, carried by a euphoria I'd never experienced.

Drugs and entertainment set inside an environment of laughter, fatherly encouragement, and empowerment. A land so unfamiliar it required a psychological passport. When I asked his help deciding on a full-time job after graduation—waitress or something more professional with benefits like my mom wanted—Dad responded, "I think you should do whichever one makes you happy," as he passed me my cone in the Dairy Queen drive-thru.

Radical.

On New Year's Eve, my junior year, Dad took me to a party. When a guy's hand crept lower on my back as we danced, his girlfriend, Brenda, tried to get him to intervene. "That guy's got his hand on your daughter's ass."

"It's her ass," Dad replied.

I felt a strange pride at his trust in me. My mom forbade concerts, assuming I'd end up getting pulled out of the mosh pit on a stretcher or found overdosed in the bathroom. She'd seen both, working security. I couldn't get my driver's license—she'd been on the scene of too many crashes.

So I rebelled, finding ways to claim my rites of passage anyway, while ricocheting between too much protection and too little.

Life settled into a smoky haze. I kept it together by taking the edge off and inhaling whatever life threw at me, and exhaling my needs. I skimmed Valium from Dad's prescription bottles, hoping it would help me chill and fill in all the gaps. I thought his return would fix everything, that his love would flood the emptiness. But it didn't.

I led a double life. On the surface, I was a straight-A student, a hard worker, bragging on Mondays about back-stage passes. Inside, I was barely holding on, breaking down from the weight of it all. My body started signaling distress, a piercing pain in my gut, breaking into a sweat as it skewered my insides. I held my breath, waiting for it to pass, hiding my discomfort under casual gestures. Nobody knew.

    I came home one afternoon to find my mother like I'd never seen her—collapsed in a dining room chair, fragile, like crumpled tissue paper. She rocked back and forth, whimpering with mumbling mixed in. I strained to hear. Her words crystallized as the heaviness of their reality tugged at a corner of my heart. "Lost the house. . ." More whimpering. "Lost the house." Tears streaked down her cheeks, something else I'd never seen.

    A wave of compassion moved my hand to her shoulder. "Shhh. . . It's okay."

    But nothing was okay.

    I tried to understand why she didn't ask to borrow money from my savings account, like with my uncle and his DUI.

    Her blank stare narrowed. "Because you said you hated me," she wailed.

    "Every teenager says that!" But what difference did any of it make now? I stood frozen inside a deal already done. I tried to absorb its impact, watching her rock and moan, her words pounding into me.

    'You said you hated me.' The world I knew faded to black once again.

---

**Core Theme / Emotional Wound:** *Survival through self-destruction.* Too much responsibility, not enough protection. When emotional pain becomes unbearable and there is no safe outlet, the body and mind seek ways to numb, rebel, and survive—even if those ways look like self-sabotage. This wound stems from feeling unseen, unsupported, and left to manage overwhelming emotions on one's own.

**Old Survival Pattern:** *Hyper-independence, secrecy, rebellion-as-coping.* Using rebellion, numbing (through substances, self-harm, emotional shutdown), and self-sabotage as a survival strategy. Acting out becomes a way to regain a sense of control or to express pain when no one is listening.

**Gut Instincts Method Stage:** *Filter.* Bombarded by chaotic messaging—parental contradictions, buried family secrets, unsafe freedom, and performative expectations. Learning (badly and brilliantly) how to filter *what is safe, what is real, and what the body knows*, even if you can't yet name it.

**Reflection:**
There's a kind of hurt that doesn't scream out loud—it leaks through choices that don't make sense from the outside. Sometimes the rebellion, the mistakes, the numbness were never really about wanting to destroy ourselves—they were desperate attempts to survive what felt unbearable.

    Maybe you know that kind of pain too. You may have learned to armor yourself in ways that once kept you safe, but now feel burdensome. It wasn't weakness. It wasn't failure. It was survival.

    What is the cost of carrying more than a child should? You stop asking for help. You become fluent in silence. And your body? It becomes the only honest narrator left.

    If you learned that, too—that silence equals survival—I see you. And I promise, there's another way.

## Reader Reflection:

1. **Self-Protective Tendencies:** Sometimes, the ways we cope with pain don't appear to be a sign of strength on the surface. However, survival itself, even through rebellion or numbness, is a testament to resilience. Where have I used rebellion—defiance, anger, acting out—as a way to protect myself when I didn't feel seen or safe?
2. **Reframing self-destruction as survival.** There's a story beneath every act of self-sabotage—a story of a heart trying to endure what felt impossible. When I look at my past patterns of self-destruction, can I see the instinct underneath them—the part of me that was trying to survive unbearable pain?
3. **Story-Supported Reflection:** Imagination can act as a balm for the spirit, particularly for children. What images or experiences do you turn to for comfort? What makes you feel safe when life feels uncertain?
4. **Reflective Visualization:** Sit quietly and try visualizing an image of peace or comfort that is personally meaningful to you. It could be a scene from childhood, a comforting presence, or even a symbol of hope.

## Affirmation:

*I release the pressure to be everything for everyone.
I claim my power, my truth, and my right to take up space.*

JENNIFER JUNIPER

Scan the Code Below to View the Video for Chapter 6:
Or go to: https://youtu.be/th4cTKYm_Yo

# Chapter 7

# Send Me an Angel

### The Angels Who Save Us
### and the Ones that Almost Destroy Us
Angels Don't Always Have Wings.

*Sometimes, angels are just ordinary people who step into our lives and remind us of what hope feels like.*
~Unknown

**Tami**

Tami appeared like a mirage, crystallizing across my scorching desert of junior year. The Thelma to my Louise—her frizzy red hair and mischievous smile a kindred spirit to my restless and uneasy heart.

We'd skip school with joints tucked in our bras and fall leaves crunching under our feet as our subconscious hummed the refrain: *We don't care about nobody, and nobody cares about us.* We climbed the rotting stairs of an abandoned house in the woods, perched on the balcony with railings deteriorated past the point of safety. That's how tough we were.

Tami hated how her body looked as much as I hated mine. When dieting didn't make us model-thin, we popped

Dexatrim and skipped lunch, smoking cigarettes instead. When deprivation didn't work, we decided to swing the other way, indulging in whatever we wanted, then sticking our fingers down our throats and purging to cancel it all out—convinced we'd found the secret.

Throwing up in a restaurant's bathroom gave me the added satisfaction of a "fuck you" to the many occasions my mom took my sister and me out to eat. *Fuck your working all the time. There's your priority, flushing down the toilet.*

Tami proposed a quick Screwdriver when I stopped to get her one morning. "Leftover booze from my parents' party," she said, motioning to the bottles on the kitchen counter.

"Breakfast of Champions!" We clinked our glasses. Alcohol's haven of heaviness kicked in quickly on an empty stomach, smoothing all the wrinkles, turning down the roar of my problems a little more with each sip.

"We've already missed most of first hour," Tami announced, as the living room clock chimed eight, "Might as well have another!"

Some kids flirted with disaster, Tami and I stuck our tongues down its throat.

Bouncing off lockers like giggly pinballs on our way to second hour, we made enough noise to get a teacher's attention. Our slurred speech earned us a three-day suspension. As the principal dialed, I relaxed into my chair safely knowing my mother unplugged the phone when she slept.

He moved on to my father's number. But discipline wasn't Dad's jurisdiction, and I was betting on a man who gave me drugs not fussing too much about me drinking vodka. (He would give me a stern few sentences about showing up to school drunk, but not about being too young to be drinking).

Mom never knew, just like when I sat across the booth from her, stoned. She didn't know that sometimes I'd skim from the bottle of gin and replace it with water. I hated the taste, but I needed the relief.

Getting away with things was better than having her love.

Tami and I drove over cliff after cliff. One night, we hitch-hiked down a dark country road to the county fair. Flirting with the carnies garnered us an invitation to their base camp later.

Their free-spiritedness danced on my skin to the point of fantasizing about running away with them. Besides the rush of hanging out on the fringe with people older than us and from places we'd never been, I felt something else amidst these misfits—a sense of belonging.

## Lonnie

With bleached strawberry-blonde hair, red pleather pants and matching red studded jacket (straight out of *Thriller*), Lonnie stood out in name *and* style. In Drama class, he'd lean over, writing notes in my planner when the teacher wasn't looking. On one Saturday, he wrote: 'Go to a party with Lonnie.' A week later: 'Have sex with Lonnie.' Rude, presumptuous, and crassly unromantic. *No way I'm giving it up to a guy fore-casting it on my calendar.*

But I sure loved parties.

When he offered me a hit of acid, I hesitated, wanting to float above it all, but scared of losing too much control. He gently cut it in half with a nail clipper on the back of a toilet. I didn't trip, but the tethers on my mind loosened enough that when he asked, 'What did you do last night?' I answered with full-on honesty.

We'd gone to my grandparents' house, and I'd said some-thing my mother didn't like. (I can't precisely recall, maybe advocating for getting my driver's license). Something in her snapped, and she jumped up and onto me, rocking the green chenille rocker, slapping me over and over again. Like she was possessed. I put my head down and my arms up in protection.

My aunt Shelly ran over to rescue me, "That's enough."

My mother turned to her and snarled, silver fang showing. "Shut up, or you're next!"

Shelly's face puzzled, unable to tell if my mother was serious. She slowly backed away, back to her seat.

Lonnie stopped blowing the blade of grass whistling between his thumbs. His look confused, then pained, strong and tender all at once, and framed with those long, curly eyelashes I was super jealous of. "She hit you?"

"Because I was sassing."

Lonnie just stared. His silence wasn't casual—it was heavy, disbelieving. I suddenly felt exposed, like I had said too much. "She shouldn't be hitting you anymore," he said again, softer, in hopes of getting through.

All I could do was stare back and blink. Dazed, I didn't know what to do with the information. So I shoved it down with everything else.

"But I was sassing," fell out of my mouth again to justify it, but it was too late. His words landed on me like a floodlight in a dark room.

## Mrs. E

On Monday morning, I asked for a pass to the guidance office. My guidance counselor had a long, hard-to-pronounce last name, so I called her Mrs. E. She always looked genuinely happy to see me: mirroring my excitement, cheerleading through all my apprehensions, or offering her office as a soft place to land on a hard day. Her long hugs gave me respite, and her squishiness and flowy dress disappeared me for a little while.

Her glasses magnified her gentle brown eyes, always interested in whatever I had to say. She listened extra intently that day. Before saying anything, she scooted her chair back from her desk, turning it to face me fully, then leaning in. "*Nothing* justifies being hit. Nothing. Not now. Not ever. I need you to understand that."

I nodded in agreement, but wondered if that was true. I sure liked the sound of it. "Nothing?"

"Nothing."

The little light of hope I tried to maintain to keep from going absolutely insane lit up a little brighter.

With each number she dialed, blood pumped harder through my veins. The pounding in my ears grew so loud that her words sounded underwater.

"I need to report the abuse of a child."

My breath caught. The pounding in my ears muffled everything else, but one thought broke through the fog: Things will get better now. We'll get the help we need.

### My English Teacher

"Your writing is excellent, Jennifer. You should be in a more challenging class." Hawk Face said. Our class nicknamed her that because her nose pointed downward, and because she was a buzzkill of a senior class advisor. With her office near Mrs. E's, I ran into her often. She pecked at me, trying to get me to transfer to AP English class whenever I saw her—like I needed more challenges.

Something in me did perk up when she said it, even timidly agreeing. It echoed the rare compliment I'd once gotten from my mother after writing thank-you cards for my confirmation gifts. She insisted on reading each one, making sure it was good enough. 'You really have a way with words, Jennifer,' she'd said, more than once.

I loved writing. It was a trait I shared with my dad and came naturally to me. English classes were my easiest; words seemed to pour out of my pen whether I was drunk, stoned, tired, or stressed.

But Hawk Face's encouragement and compliments didn't brush me with the softness of feathers or instill in me the steely confidence of an apex predator. Transferring to AP English presented a level I didn't dare rise to for fear of wobbling my high GPA.

I threw every rock of an excuse at her I could. "I'll think about it. I'm struggling with Trig right now." Or, "I'll talk to you about it later. I've got my hands full with the play." (*Full* was a bit of an exaggeration. I had a couple of lines).

How could I straddle my two worlds of good student and bad girl if I took an advanced class? *What if I'm not good enough?* An easy 'A' was the better choice. I doubled down on my double life with each excuse.

Even though I didn't take up the challenge, the offering was everything to me. It threw a lifeline to my fledgling self-esteem, and I clung to it when the seas got rough.

### Brenda

Dad's new girlfriend wasn't like his other flames. No heavy makeup, no drama, and eyes that widened with interest and concern as she listened. She tracked my life from weekend to weekend and became a friend. A maternal presence filling in the unconditional love void I kept tripping over and falling through.

# GUT INSTINCTS

She noticed when I winced and rubbed my belly to soothe the cramping. My signature loquaciousness choked off and restricted to nods, shakes, and 'mm-hm's.' The episodes were coming more frequently, and the spasms had turned savage. My digestive system didn't seem to like most foods. It would struggle as if pushing it through a passage too small. I pictured my intestines like a hose with a kink in it. The pain seemed to be growing right along with me.

In a moment alone, grabbing snacks from the kitchen, Brenda and her big, brown, caring eyes asked. "Are you feeling okay?"

My knee-jerk response was that I was fine. Fine. "I'm fine." I turned so my eyes wouldn't give me away.

She saw right through it. "I had awful stomach aches when I was your age."

I lowered my guard a little, my words cautiously venturing out. "You did?"

She described symptoms like mine: hot, poking pain, feverish flushes and sweats, nausea, the explosive, extra-embarrassing gas. I was no longer a lone freak. My guard lowered inside her empathy.

"What did they do about it?" Desperation for some kind of a solution dripped off my every word.

Brenda's weak coffee eyes turned espresso. Her lids blinked back the memory as her words poured on, telling the story of a colonoscopy gone wrong—waking up with a tube winding through her intestines and being denied more anesthesia with a doctor's dismissive, 'We're almost done.'

I gasped. Whatever trusting part of me had peeked its head out scurried back inside and slammed the door. *No way am I volunteering for that!*

Her story stayed on me like black smoke. I tucked my secret back inside and buried it even deeper.

# JENNIFER JUNIPER

**Theme / Emotional Wound:** *Being seen without shame. Yearning for safe connection.* The tender tension between:
- Wanting to be known and cared for
- Fearing what that visibility might cost
- Beginning to test what safety feels like with others

The wound isn't only abandonment—it's having *no consistent reflection of your worth*. Each "angel" reflects a tiny glimmer of it. This is *emergent hope*, raw and necessary.

**Old Survival Pattern:** *Hiding pain* while testing closeness; craving care but *expecting abandonment*; confusing attention with danger.

**Gut Instincts Stage:** *Feel* (with glimmers of *Face* and *Filter*) Learning to feel what it means to be seen. Testing your inner *Filter*: Is this safe? Is this true? And start facing what hurts when you let someone in.

**Reflection:**
Sometimes, the people who change everything don't save you in one sweeping gesture—they show up in fragments. A word. A glance. A moment of seeing you when no one else did.

    I didn't call them angels back then. But now I know they were. Each one handed me a mirror. And in each one, I saw a part of myself worth keeping.

    Maybe you've had people like that. Perhaps you've been that mirror for someone else. Either way, you are part of something bigger now—the quiet, unstoppable ways healing finds us.

**Reader Reflection:**

1. **Story-Supported Reflection:** What have past experiences of loneliness taught you about yourself? How has that impacted your relationships today?
2. **Your Early Angels:** Who are the people who first saw your pain or truth, without judgment? What did it feel like to be witnessed without needing to perform or explain?

    Sometimes the hardest thing to trust is our potential. When have you shrank from an opportunity, a challenge, a moment of growth—because you were afraid you wouldn't be able to sustain it or feared being exposed as "not enough"?

## Affirmation:

*I am worthy of being seen and still safe.
It is okay to let the light in one mirror at a time.
I receive care without condition.*

Scan the Code Below to View the Video for Chapter 7:
Or go to: https://youtu.be/nZFhJ5VeoEo

## JENNIFER JUNIPER

———————————————

By the end of Part One, you'll see your struggles as intel rather than problems to fix, and begin recognizing the patterns that have been running beneath the surface.

———————————————

# Part Two

# Reconnection

## The Art Of Deep Listening

*Transformation begins when we move from opposition to collaboration with our inner intelligence*

# Chapter 8

# Hell Is For Children

### Breaking the Chain of Generational Trauma
Approval equals love, performance establishes worth, rebellion and self-harm help you survive.

*My pain does not define me.
I am worthy of love, safety, and healing,
no matter what I've been told.*

"Where are your bruises if you're so abused?" Grandma asked, voice sneering, eyes ice-cold. Her words pinned my sister and me to the entryway, making us grip our little suitcases and uncertainties tighter. She snorted with disdain. What did I expect from a woman who kept a flyswatter balanced atop the kitchen phone in easy reach for spanking butts as much as swatting flies?

*Why didn't the social worker take us to Dad's place?* I wondered for the millionth time.

She sat in her chair against the dining room wall, in a straight-on view of the door. And it was *her* chair; anyone sitting there would vacate it immediately if she made any towards it. (She would say, 'Oh, don't get up,' but you knew better.) From that throne she ruled the house, with the

## JENNIFER JUNIPER

whole first floor in view, and the second one accessed by yelling up the staircase to her left.

Grandma was not the stereotypical hugging, doting, bragging about her grandkids type. When the church pastor came over to discuss the annual tithing commitment, she brazenly wore her slip to the appointment (with her girdle underneath). Being heavyset made her all the more intimidating.

Her customers at the bakery thought she was as sweet as the confections she sold them, but they didn't hear her mutter behind their backs before the bell on the door stopped tinkling their exit. "Did you see how short her skirt was? Floosie." "I hope she doesn't eat any of that cake; those pants are too tight already."

It stressed me to be in the middle of her two radically different personas, their sole witness, the keeper of another secret. I felt the pain of her insults, even when directed at someone else. I couldn't explain it, and I couldn't escape it. When it happened at closer range around the kitchen table, and her target was Grandpa, that pain became even more acute.

Grandpa was one of the two people I felt loved by un-con-di-tion-al-ly. (The other one was my other grandpa.) As a little girl, I'd spend Sunday afternoons squeezed into his recliner, munching popcorn from a paper grocery bag and watching endless football. Summers, we'd swap that for fishing and my squealing as I tried to get a worm on my hook. Grandpa would take over, laughing and saving me. I squealed again when a bite tugged my line. He'd move behind me, circling me in his strong, hairy arms to help reel it in.

Watching helplessly as Grandma berated my super kind, ever-patient, often clowning Grandpa over an entire Sunday dinner distressed me even more. He never fought back—as much as I willed him to with my eyes: *Say something! Don't let her talk to you like that*! He just winked at me his usual *Don't worry.*

Had I known that telling Mrs. E. would lead me there, I would've kept my mouth shut.

I tried to build a we're-in-this-together team with my sister, but she just kept whining to go home. "Why did you have to say anything!? This is even worse." Watery blue eyes reflecting her and Mom's team color.

I spent the weekend dodging Grandma's emotional landmines and fantasizing about getting adopted so I could escape the family entirely. Sunday evening, the social worker called.

"Lisa can go home, but not you." Grandma held me in her narrow, icy gaze. "Your mother said you're the one causing all the problems." Her tone reflected agreement.

That night, I slept on a bed of loneliness and confusion. *Am I the only one who sees what's wrong with this family?* I silent screamed. Something inside me cracked from the reverberation. I'd been punished before, but this was different. This was exile. I wasn't being grounded or scolded, more like discarded—for telling the truth.

My stomach churned, tightening into knots so hard I curled into myself.

A few days later, the call came that I could go home, but the weekend of rejection had pushed me farther away. The next day, I threw a few things in a bag and ran away to a friend's house. The cops came for me and took me home. The pressure would build again, and I'd find another friend's house to crash at. Again, the cops brought me back. I'd sulk past the officer and Mom, chatting like friends in the driveway.

"Hi, Debbie. Hi, Ron."

"Hi, Steve. Hey, Debbie."

## JENNIFER JUNIPER

She admonished me from my bedroom doorway, "I work with them, Jennifer. Do you know how this makes me look?"

Heat filled my veins. I held back my yell. *Do you only care about how things **look**? Don't you care about how I **feel**?!*

I counted down the days to freedom, like hash marks a prisoner makes on the wall of their cell. Hedged my bets like a savvy gambler, placing an equal stack of chips on rebelling and excelling. In my outside world, I moved with the masses: seniors doing typical senior year stuff—cap and gown, searching "For Rent" ads, figuring out what we wanted to do with our lives.

On the inside, the stakes were much higher. I curated perfection, as evidenced by arguing my scores in Economics class. Often. (So often, it was mentioned on more than one occasion by those signing my yearbook: 'I'll miss you arguing your score in Econ.')

'98' glared from the top of the page, taunting me. I began madly flipping through the returned assignment to see the red marks indicating what I'd gotten wrong. Seeing none, I shot my hand up. "Why didn't I get 100? You didn't mark anything wrong."

"No paper is perfect," the teacher tried to shut me down and move on.

After a few rounds of back and forth between us, my classmates would groan and mumble that I still got an 'A' and should be happy. They didn't understand. I *needed* that '100.'

When I missed the mark, or when sedating with drugs, sex, and alcohol wasn't enough—or I couldn't escape by running away—I escaped *in*. Going to my jewelry box, I lifted out the red felt earring insert and pushed aside the bracelets, uncovering the razor blades stashed there. Ever so delicately, I carried them to the bathroom. Ceremoniously.

It was, strangely, a sacred act.

# GUT INSTINCTS

Slicing into its milky white, my wrist responded with a garnet bead. I watched it swell until it slid over the side and dropped onto the white porcelain sink with a starburst splat.

*Splat.*

*Splat.*

Cutting dropped all my sadness and stress into slow motion, making it a more morose and all-consuming version that I could sink into like a warm bath. The deeper I cut, the quieter everything became—except for the gnawing ache in my gut.

Riding the line between life and death released me as I softly sang the theme song from *M*A*S*H* that I'd learned to play on the piano. *Suicide is painless; it brings on many changes, and I can take or leave it if I please.*

It was a pain that had rules, followed a rhythm. It made sense. A pain I could stop.

It infused me with the power I needed to hold on a bit longer, just until graduation. *I can move out the very next day.* I pictured it over and over again: packing up my stuff and saying goodbye to the evil regime where I didn't feel heard, accepted, or even loved.

Like Dorothy, I dreamed of a better life over the rainbow. But I was running out of song.

---

**Theme / Emotional Wound:** *Betrayal + Exile from Belonging.* This chapter is about being punished not for doing wrong, but for telling the truth. It's the psychic fracture of being cast out for exposing the very thing that's hurting you.

**Old Survival Pattern:** *Perfectionism as a plea for worth.* Self-harm as sacred control. Navigating rejection by dissocia-ting inward or excelling outward.

**Gut Instincts Healing Method Stage:** *Face.* The peak of facing—the family's gaslighting, the system's ineptitude, the gap between appearances and reality. The body is not just holding the pain, but mirroring the pain with flares, cramping, and the private rituals of harm.

---

**Reflection:**
Sometimes, the deepest pain isn't from what happens to us—but what doesn't happen after. No comfort. No validation. No rescue. When no one stands up for your truth, your body stands up for it instead.

Maybe you've carried pain so quietly that even you started to forget how loud it was. Perhaps you learned to carry grief so silently that it began to sound normal.

If so, know this: you were never meant to survive this alone. You deserve to be heard. You were born to be seen. You are allowed to ask for more. You were meant to rise.

**Reader Reflection:**

1. **Identify Safe Connections.** List the people in your life who provide unconditional support and respect for your boundaries. Consider what safety truly looks and feels like for you. What steps can you take to cultivate this feeling in your life?
2. **Reflect on Your Angels.** Who has shown up in your life during challenging times? Identify the "angels" who offered perspective or support, even if it was hard to accept their help at first. What did these individuals reveal about your personal strength?

# GUT INSTINCTS

3. **Explore Feelings Around Being Seen.** Sometimes, like with a counselor or teacher, being truly seen is both liberating and intimidating. Reflect on what it means to be seen for who you are—vulnerabilities and strengths alike.

## Affirmation:

*My truth matters, even when others refuse to hear it.
I am worthy of love, safety, and healing—now and always.*

Scan the Code Below to View the Video for Chapter 8:
Or go to: https://youtu.be/zViZ4Ra9tTg

# Chapter 9

# Into The Mystic

### Awakening to Your True Nature
Where self-discovery meets the spiritual,
and we remember we are more than we thought.

*The only journey is the one within.*
~Rainer Maria Rilke

The summer before my senior year granted me two long-term wishes: gaining freedom from my mother and getting closer to my dad. I'd been begging her to let me go live with him, and she finally acquiesced in her typical cynical tone, sure I'd see my *real* father, the same jerk she saw.

"He doesn't even have a bedroom for you. You'll have to sleep on the couch."

Was she trying to temper my expectations? Impossible. Everything I'd been dying to have happen was happening. What did I care what I'd be sleeping on?

Stepping through his doorway to stay, I exhaled a breath I didn't even realize I was holding. Gone were the parental expectations of perfection—I could be myself. Dad thought everything I did was a reflection of me, not him. I was off-leash. Freedom and the ability to make my own decisions fostered a sense of agency over my life. The more choices I made, the more empowered I felt.

I experimented with identities and ideals a lot that summer.

Eating along with Dad's diabetic diet, I lost weight. Skinless chicken breasts. Chamomile tea before bed. Nilla Wafers the sugariest thing in his cupboard. I almost liked how I looked.

*Almost.*

The vice grip around my waist loosened right along with my jeans. I don't know if it was the eating or the ease, but when I open the mental scrapbook from that summer, there's no painful belly memorabilia on any of the pages.

I reveled in my new experience of family, even though Dad constantly introduced me to people who were shocked to meet me. 'I had no idea Michael had a daughter!' The common refrain didn't bother me at all. I enjoyed being a surprise—Dad and I were an act again! I was agog at how gorgeous, talented, and gregarious everyone I met was. I became ensconced in his ever-widening social circle of coolness—drummers, dancers, producers, and sound engineers.

Besides, I graded Dad as generously as he graded me. I held Mom to the same high standards she had for me.

Dad and I shared a crazed love for Prince. At Mom's house, a cardboard cutout of Prince on his purple motorcycle stood in the corner of my bedroom, positioned so I could fall asleep under his watchful eye—after kissing him goodnight, of course. It was a record store display to promote the release of the *Purple Rain* soundtrack, and Dad asked his owner friend if he could have it when the campaign ended.

A year and a half later, MTV was gearing up for the world premiere of the video for Prince's new single: *Raspberry Beret.* [Back in the day, MTV used to show music videos. Radical, I know.] World premieres meant the video first played at 10:00 pm and again every hour on the hour for twenty-four hours.

Problem was, the grocery store where I worked as a bagger closed at 10:00. I was so worried I'd miss the premiere that I sent up a quick little prayer while dropping Frosted Flakes into a bag. At 9:55, with the store empty, I asked if I could leave a little early. Then I ran the whole way home—pumping my arms across two huge parking lots—bursting through the apartment door in a sweet summer sweat.

"I've got it ready!" Dad yelled from the living room. His typically deep voice rose to a fevered pitch of anticipation.

There he was, wheeled in front of the small television, remote in hand, an excited smile mirroring mine. And there I was, basking in the connection that comes from sharing something you love so much with someone who loves it as much as you do. I felt seen. Known. In that living room, with that video playing, rocking out and singing along with my dad, I belonged. Finally. Just like I always dreamed I would.

I slept in fifty-five-minute increments that night: watching, singing, dancing, then swooning onto the couch and setting my alarm for the top of the hour to do it all over again.

*Mom would never let me do this.*

When the world ended because some guy broke my heart, Dad pulled from the famous feminist Gloria Steinem to help me put it in perspective. 'A woman without a man is like a fish without a bicycle.'

I finally learned how to drive. Without the pressure to do it perfectly, I picked it up quickly. My mother had taken me out twice. After being scolded for making too many mistakes, I was so stressed that I practiced with some friends to get better. The next time out, she chastised me for being too good and interrogated me about who I'd practiced with.

## JENNIFER JUNIPER

I couldn't seem to find the sweet spot for Mom's approval—a moving target taped to a cheetah that was also a shape-shifter. Seemed easier to lay down my bow and arrow and resort to asking friends for rides.

Dad was going down his own new road—spirituality. Having maxed out all the benefits traditional medicine had to offer, he sought relief beyond valium's reach and set off in search of more esoteric modalities.

Around his neck, he wore a crocheted pouch filled with crystals meant to infuse his ailments with healing energy. The nerves in his unusable legs still delivered stabbing pains, randomly and quite unfairly. On good days, I watched in awe as my father whizzed around corners, tipped up on one side—or balanced on back wheels, chatting away, laughing, and looking like his cool, usual self, with the addition of fingerless black leather gloves.

On bad days, his head hung low, hair stringy and smelly, mustache drooping, giving away the frown that hid beneath. He was quiet on those days, brooding and moody—somewhere else, even though he sat right next to me.

The second Sunday of the month, Dad took me to a psychic fair, where he looked to powers beyond this world for relief amidst mandala tapestries and the celestial scents of sage and patchouli. A tarot card reader revealed the strong character traits I could count on to help me navigate the world, and for someone who'd only just met me, asked eerily accurate questions about the challenges I was facing.

As an early birthday present, Dad paid an astrologer to do my birth chart. It highlighted the positive attributes I was born with, as well as the planets that were in play at the time of my birth and the elements that influenced me.

All of it described me more accurately than I could've described myself. Character traits such as... *appearing strong and compassionate to those who look to you for support and strength. This may occasionally mask your insecurities and prevent you from seeking help from others.*

Other pieces were easier to hear. *Sun conjunct Neptune natives are psychically sensitive, emotional, sentimental, poorly understood people driven by romantic ideals. Dreamers who will either become a Don Quixote, or with wisdom, a messiah. Masters of their own minds.*

The astrologer concluded with a summation that filled me with gratitude and hope. "The good things that have happened to you aren't by luck, but by design. And there's more to come."

The fringe of the purple crushed velvet tapestry dangling over his table tickled my knee as I drank in his words and got even more excited for my future.

I'd gone to the fair because I happily tagged along to whatever Dad planned. I hadn't anticipated seeing myself in a new light that would elevate my self-esteem, or seeing God in a myriad of ways that would expand my access. I carried the nascent sense of self and divinity with me as we left, protecting it like one would a budding flower in a thunderstorm.

Back at my dad's place, I poked around his bookcase, hoping to further my indoctrination beyond the limits of dogma to the fertile soil of *Be Here Now*. Its prismatic cover and elegant gold pages with wild patterns were unlike any book I'd seen. It read more like a scroll with little vignettes that stood alone rather than following the plot of a proper story—a picture book for adults.

The author sounded wise, but also full of childlike exuberance. Most of it flew over my head. But on one essential part, I agreed wholeheartedly: 'The Bible is not a metaphor. It's not a story made up to teach us how to be moral beings.

It's a straight message of how it is when man lives in the spirit, and the spirit is right inside... The whole game is based on faith.'

My exuberance kicked in. *I knew it!*

I knew Ram Dass's proclamation to be true from personal experience—faith was indeed the access point. I thought about my dad suddenly gaining six more inches of non-paralyzed muscle after waking up from a coma. I went further back to the scene in the grass, where the orchestrated comfort was so big and strong that it calmed my crying and kept me company as I walked the world with a Dad-shaped space by my side.

Such monumental moments surpassed the capabilities of mere mortals and were trademarks of a power coming from someplace beyond. Reading Ram Dass's stream of consciousness added ballast to my budding supernatural ideology.

*The Little Prince* made things much easier to grasp, illustrating the search for meaning in kid-level terms, with talking animals. A fox saying, *It's only with the heart that one can see rightly; what is essential is invisible to the eye.* A little prince advocating for the child-like qualities of curiosity and dismissing adults' way of seeing because they lacked imagin*ation* and *were often wrong.*

I knew this feeling intimately. My sister and I once got the bedtime giggles so bad (from reading the book *Bedtime Giggles*) that we upset our mom. The more we tried to stop the worse our giggles got, and the more our mom told us to control them—confusing our young minds. It felt so good to laugh until you cried and your belly ached. And giggles don't exactly have an on/off switch.

My heart yearned for adulthood, but the prince had a point. I incorporated his emphasis on exploring one's inner and outer world into my toolbox. The world softened a little that day.

Competitive Me went on summer vacation as well, relaxing outside of the performance pressure cooker. In my father's world of creative types, they were all about self-expression and individuality, so I stopped trying to blend in and played around with my style and unique stamp on the world.

Who was I when I wasn't trying to be someone else?

I sprouted in this new soil. Nowhere was this more evident than when I went against the big hair style of the 80s. Perms had been my go-to ever since age eleven, when I huddled under an old bath towel as my first home perm burned my nostrils, eyes, and throat. (Who wouldn't want more of that!)

Dad treated me to the avant-garde salon where he went. I flipped through the style books while we waited in red leather chairs, surrounded and inspired by the Art Deco style of the place.

I picked out a daring, asymmetrical cut.

Frizzes of a worn-out perm sprinkled the floor, and I looked at them like parts of my personality—clippings of, and freedom from, the fatherless version of me I no longer wanted to be. I could make such a bold move because I anchored in myself. The deep emotional connection with my dad mended the feelings of isolation and inadequacy I harbored. Tethered to his love and acceptance, I fearlessly dove into new ideas and experimented with my style.

Something bloomed inside me while I was living with my dad that summer. I aligned more with joy and authenticity. Getting my driver's license, weighing in on decisions that affected me, and being trusted to handle more freedom—in one summer, I gained the ground I'd been losing for years and caught up to my peers.

My whole emotional landscape shifted—joy, expansion, laughter, and ease, feeling valued, free, connected. Safe.

---

**Theme / Emotional Wound:** *Emergence of self / First taste of emotional freedom.* This chapter explores what it means to finally feel emotionally safe enough to explore identity, spirituality, and self-expression. It's a moment of profound *relief* and *reclamation*.

**Old Survival Pattern:** *Over-adapting, perfectionism, shrinking to be safe.* Constant monitoring and adjusting for approval leaves little room to discover who you actually are beneath the performance.

**Gut Instincts Healing Method Stage:** *Free.* This is the essence of the *Free* stage. Not only making your own decisions—you're inhabiting yourself, and you're discovering your capacity to connect joyfully rather than survive reactively.

**Reflection:**
Sometimes healing doesn't look like a breakthrough. It looks like a summer—a summer where you forget to measure yourself. Where you let your laughter be too loud, your hunger be too real, your curiosity be too much.

A summer where you try on new ways of being, not because you have to fix yourself, but because you are finally free to explore.

Maybe that's what real safety is: space without conditions. Space where your body isn't bracing for impact. A space where you can breathe without asking permission.

And maybe that season of becoming is already unfolding inside you.

**Reader Reflection:**

1. **Reclaiming Power and Control:** In what ways do you feel powerless in your life today, and how does that connect to your past experiences? What small actions can you take to regain a sense of control in areas where you feel stuck or overwhelmed?
2. **Dreaming of Freedom:** Have you ever longed for freedom from a situation, environment, or relationship? What steps can you take today to create more freedom in your life—physically, emotionally, or spiritually? What does your version of "over the rainbow" look like, and how can you take small steps toward that vision?
3. **Resilience and Hope:** Despite the hardships you've faced, what inner strengths have helped you survive and keep going?

    What gives you hope now, and how can you nurture that hope as part of your healing journey?

## Affirmation:

*I am free to evolve beyond who I was told to be.*
*I am safe enough to expand, express, and belong to myself.*
*I carry joy in my bones, and it is sacred.*

JENNIFER JUNIPER

Scan the Code Below to View the Video for Chapter 9:
Or go to: https://youtu.be/03JU9YLCDL4

## Chapter 10

# Another Brick In The Wall
### (Pt. 1, 2, & 3)

**The Paradox of Self-Protection**
What we build to keep pain out
often keeps healing from getting in.

*The walls we build to protect ourselves sometimes end up trapping us in the very pain we're trying to escape.*
~Brene Brown

After a summer of freedom and feeling like myself for the first time, returning home for my senior year felt like stepping back into a straitjacket—each day tighter than the last.

No one in my family liked my new haircut, but their opinions didn't weigh nearly as heavily as they used to. In the yearbook where everyone sported a massive halo of permed curls and bangs that shot skyward, I stood out as a layered, gel-crunchy statement of self. Not just a middle finger to conformity, but a quiet confidence that lived in my smile, in the softness of my eyes.

I wasn't rebelling. I was becoming.

You can see it in my eyes—not knowing exactly where I was going, but confident I'd get there. It was the look of a girl who had her father *and* a foothold, no longer looking to attach herself to someone—*anyone*—like a barnacle.

Back in the slammer after my summer reprieve, the backfiring of my mother's plan made tensions between us even worse. I dodged her as much as I could. Dancing around her schedule was easy—she worked second shift, and I worked every day after school at Grandma's bakery. Mom would be at work when I came home, and I'd already be deep in dreams when she returned.

She always called home once, randomly, sometime after curfew. Not to ask how my day was or how Lisa had fared on the test she was anxious about, but to make sure we were home—like some remote warden. We always were, and so were some of our friends. Since we couldn't stay out with them, they'd come home with us, and when the phone rang, a hush fell on the room, right on cue. (My sister finally trusted my way of doing things.)

After everyone left, we'd smooth some of the footprints out of the carpet but not too many, or we'd trigger an interrogation about what we were trying to cover up. We learned the hard way *never* to vacuum, way too suspicious.

Mother's presence left souvenirs—a towel hanging to dry, the smell of Chanel No. 5 when she'd been on a date. But in reality, I lived in a ghost town. Two people passing through a house that never felt like home, clashing only when our schedules collided, like sparks in a powder keg.

I'd throw things in a bag and run to a friend's house before the sulfur smell cleared. We couldn't seem to move past our opposing stances of 'I can't trust you' and 'How do you know if you never give me a chance!'

I'd scream-write in my journal sometimes, about her reining me in while I strained to ride alongside my peers. *Perfect grades aren't enough. It's like she wants me to be a perfect person!! I can't be. No one can. Come on, I'm seventeen, I'm supposed to be figuring it out and making mistakes. It's like a test I can't pass no matter how hard I try.*

Journaling helped me process my past more astutely, turning over rocks and reliving experiences, ready to leave it all behind yet still trying to make sense of it. I couldn't go to the RATT concert with my friends because it 'wasn't safe,' but I'd spent a summer being a full-time babysitter to some kids from church—barely younger than me—whose dad suddenly moved out. Nobody asked me, and I didn't get paid. My age is vague, but I remember making chocolate pudding in a blender, scraping the sides while it was whirring, and shooting brown sweetness up to the ceiling like a geyser.

Further proof that permissions weren't granted out of maturity, but convenience.

"I feel like a pawn in my own life." I huffed to Janette, my friend and savior, who suggested the savvy workaround of a sleepover the night of the concert.

"You have all these restrictions, but no one home to enforce them." She wisely observed.

"She only sees the dangers in everything and uses them to control me. I can't wait to move out." My freedom loomed over the horizon, glistening like the Land of Oz.

More and more, my family appeared like a circus to me. I'd trapeze between my mother's overparenting and my father's liberal leniency, wanting more from the parent who wanted little time with me and less from the one who suffocated me. I walked the tightrope between being a straight-A student and a girl trying everything to dull the pain and gain more control over her life.

At my bakery job, I'd make out with boys in the stockroom. Starved for love and affection, I gave my body to anyone who wanted it. Balancing on the edge of the counter and wrapping my legs around their waist for torque, as the black hole inside me sucked them in deeper and deeper, desperate for someone to get close enough, to want me so much they'd fill the aching emptiness.

But no one ever did.

When fights widened the chasm between Mom and me, or Dad canceled our weekend plans, I'd tuck even further into myself, stressing about my tummy and stressing about my mind that wasn't that healthy either.

At least the intense stomachaches came and went, but the pull to the dark side was incessant.

It all got the better of me one day. Unable to hold on—exhausted from trying to be heard, aggravated by watching my friends blow by me with more privileges while I stayed home, or risked getting caught 'disobeying'—I reached for my valium stash. I wasn't sure if it was enough to kill me, but at that moment I didn't care. I just wanted the pain to stop.

Fear gripped me and pulled me a little closer with each minute ticking by in first period. *What if it is enough?* I didn't want to die. I just couldn't keep living this way. Terror swallowed me whole, and I tapped out by asking for a pass to the guidance office. With tears streaming down my cheeks, I confessed to Mrs. E. and begged her to help me. She held my hand as she called the ambulance, squeezing it periodically to reassure me that everything would be okay. That was her role, talking me down off the ledge.

They wheeled me out of school on a stretcher.

I hadn't even stopped vomiting when my mother arrived, apologized to the nurse for my behavior, and announced that no further care would be necessary. "She's just doing this for attention." As soon as my stomach emptied, she ordered, "Get dressed. We're leaving." Brushing off the doctor's recommendation to stay overnight for observation and a full psych eval in the morning.

I leaned my head against the window on the drive home. Once again, help was right there, but I couldn't have it.

*I just need to make it to graduation.*

To Mom, running away was rebellion but to me, it was salvation. I couldn't cut anymore—my sister was so upset when she found my razor blades, she took them and made me promise I'd never do it again. I knew from the valium overdose that I didn't want to die, so suicide was out. I couldn't drink when I needed to function; the school suspension had taught me that. I couldn't live with my dad and go to the same school. He also hadn't offered.

Running away was the only solution.

Sometime during my last semester, Mom sent word via my sister that she wouldn't chase me anymore. Ironic, since I hadn't gone far. Just two apartment buildings down, sharing a friend's room and her family, who felt more like family than mine.

Graduation was a semi-normal moment. Dad smiled bigger than I'd ever seen him, bigger than the night of the Prince video premiere. Both my parents were in the same vicinity again, so we almost looked normal. They stayed a distance apart in some subconscious agreement, I assumed. I wondered, as I'd wondered a million times before, how they ever got together in the first place.

I once asked my dad, and the opening of the Journey song "Don't Stop Believin'" played in my head as he told the story.

*Just a small-town girl, livin in a lonely world* (helping raise all those siblings and working at Dairy Queen), *she took the midnight train going anywhere. Just a city boy, born and raised in South Detroit* (he'd proposed to her from a phone booth there). *He took the midnight train going anywhere.*

After graduating from my same high school, my army-brat dad—born in Japan—followed my grandpa to his next orders in Michigan. He called her one day and opened with, "What would you say if I were wearing platform shoes, had hair down to my ass, and was in a rock-n-roll band?"

"I could change you." She replied.

At seventeen, I had zero marriage experience, but that sounded like a bad way to start one. "And you married her anyway?"

He shrugged. "I thought I needed changing."

As I stood there in cap and gown, honor cord draped around my neck, I couldn't shake the thought that this rite of passage was more beginning than end. For a night I had the same curfew as my friends, making me *feel* normal for a change.

The clanging bell of liberation rang louder in the following days as I packed up my stuff—including cardboard Prince—and broke out of my childhood house of pain. The capricious control and impossible-to-please rein were over. I dove excitedly, wholeheartedly, into my own apartment. My dad cosigned—I wasn't an adult until November. (Oh, but I felt like one!) With no one reigning over me but me, it felt more like a castle.

But echoes of home haunted its hallways.

The motto of our graduating class turned out to be an apt personal slogan as well. 'What lies behind us and what lies before us are tiny matters compared to what lies within us.' The quote from Emerson was also foreboding. My internal striving picked up where my mother's prodding left off, drowning out the sound of my body breaking down even more.

## GUT INSTINCTS

Any meal could become a battle. My gut sometimes moaned warnings at the mere sight of food, 'Dooooon't eeeeeeven eeeeeeat.' It groaned like an alien as it digested.

I began to notice that in moving out, I'd packed up things I didn't intend to. The word "stupid" would speak itself in my head when I made a simple mistake, like cutting my finger open while slicing lemons at work. I had a bad habit of hurling brutal insults at myself whenever I was late (which was often), or when my car slid off an icy road and got stuck in a ditch (which was common in Wisconsin winters). Sometimes when I opened my mouth, my mother would come out.

I hadn't only packed it all up—I'd swallowed it.

That explained the pain in my belly, gaining force and sharpness. The food scraped its way through my intestines like it had corners. At times, it would stop traveling altogether, like hitting a wall—gurgling and bloating me as if things were backing up. Digestion hurt going the right direction, but boy did it hurt like hell going the wrong way.

I said nothing about it to anyone. I lied at work, saying I'd been in the bathroom for so long because I was cleaning it. I would hold in the gas—its release could go on forever and smelled like rotting sewage—until the sharp pains and bloating became unbearable, sending me outside for some "fresh air" followed by quizzical looks as I opened the door to Wisconsin's frigid winter.

Or I'd light a cigarette whether I wanted to or not, frantically rummaging through my purse in a race against the bubbles painfully stretching my bowels as they moved closer to the exit, hoping to light one in time to mask the putrid stench and evade my company's horrified looks.

I suffered alone, broken and ashamed. Different. Still stuck on the outside, trying to find my way in.

# JENNIFER JUNIPER

---

**Theme / Emotional Wound:** *Internalized oppression and the illusion of freedom.* This chapter explores the painful realization that even after escaping external control, the voices of shame, perfectionism, and self-harm live on inside the body.

**Old Survival Pattern:** Overachieving to outrun pain, self-criticism as inherited language, and emotional suppression through independence. *Freedom on the outside, but captivity inside.*

**Gut Instincts Healing Method Stage:** *Feel → Filter → Face* (all three intersect). This is where the method *converges*—your body is screaming, your mind is filtering, and your soul is facing what survival has cost. It's the moment when emotional awareness begins to press against somatic truth.

**Reflection:**
We all build walls. Sometimes the bricks are obvious—grief, betrayal, abandonment. Sometimes they're harder to name—an absent look, a sharp word, a hand that never reached back.
    And sometimes, the ones who hurt us were the same ones we depended on to survive.
    I thought leaving the house would be enough to leave the war behind. But trauma doesn't stay in the places where it happened. It travels. It gets woven into your thoughts, your self-talk, your digestion, your breath.
    That's the thing about trauma: it doesn't live in the past—it lives in the body. And you can't outrun what you've swallowed.

# GUT INSTINCTS

**Reader Reflection:**

1. **Listening to the Body:** How do you respond when your body sends you signals of distress or discomfort? What steps could you take to better care for your physical and emotional well-being?
2. **The Desire to Be Seen and Heard:** Reflect on a time when you felt invisible or unheard. How did you express that need, and how was it received? What's one way you can better honor your voice and needs today?
3. **Resilience in Adversity:** When faced with challenging or painful situations, how do you cope? Are there ways you can turn to yourself for strength and healing rather than external sources that may not serve you?
4. **Spiritual Curiosity:** What role does spirituality or curiosity about the unseen play in your healing journey? Are there books, practices, or experiences (like the psychic fairs) that have opened new doors for you?

## Affirmation:

*I am allowed to unlearn what hurt me.*
*I don't owe anyone my silence.*

JENNIFER JUNIPER

Scan the Code Below to View the Video for Chapter 10:
Or go to: https://youtu.be/R71mJwIKKwA

# Chapter 11

# Go Your Own Way

### The Power of Choice
True direction comes from turning down the volume
on others' voices and tuning into your own.

*No one saves us but ourselves.*
*No one can and no one may.*
*We ourselves must walk the path.*
~Buddha

I broke out of my small hometown into the big city next door, Madison—Wisconsin's capital and a college town. I might've made my own decision to continue my education, but before I ever reached the age where one looks that far down the road, I was told that college was where it led.

"Fine," I answered. "I'll go to Cosmetology School." The stained faces on all my Barbies, courtesy of marker makeup, attested to my passion. They'd been to the beauty salon so many times that their hair was shorter than Ken's.

"That's not college." Mom quipped, her tone slicing through my excitement like a razor through stubble.

"Sure it is. Says so right here." I pointed to the brochure from the guidance office.

She shot me that look—the one that repeated her words for her.

I didn't have a backup passion. So I chose Business School because 'business' meant 'money,' and money made my mother happy. She gave her blessing.

It didn't matter in the end, because I never went—a no-show to my own future. I had a sneaking suspicion I wasn't the business school type. I didn't know what type I was, but I reasoned that graduating younger than my peers afforded me a buffer of time to figure it out without falling behind. I decided to keep waitressing at the diner, building up my bank account since I'd be footing the bill.

A homeless woman came in almost daily. She stayed for hours, ordering only Diet Coke and wet naps, asking for refills on both, and took a spongebath in her booth. She paid with sticky coins scattered across the table. No tip. We'd cringe when she walked in, drawing straws for who had to take her.

But as winter crept in, and I grew up a little, the mocking gave way to worry. *It's November, how does she stay warm?* Her refuge was a red vinyl booth—mine had been my older boyfriend's apartment above the adult bookstore Red Letter News. I knew what it was like to live on the outskirts of normalcy and feel the sting of others' judgments.

Empathy stirred within me and I could no longer join my co-workers in making fun. The next time someone reached for the straws, I put out my hand out to stop them and said, "I'll take her," surprising everyone, including myself. Acknowledging her resilience gave me glimpses into my own. I'd been through a lot, maybe she had, too, and we were both still here doing the best we could with what we had.

A few weeks later, I put my throbbing feet up on my secondhand coffee table—nylons discarded and stuck to themselves where mayonnaise (or something) had dried—

and reached again for the college catalog. I leafed through it with all the seriousness of searching for a new shade of nail polish in Cosmo. A turn of the page revealed a degree titled Human Services. Something in me surged towards it.

*I bet that's what Laura had.*

You get a caseworker like Laura when you get busted for shoplifting at fourteen, and the judge offers you the option of a psych eval instead of a fine and a criminal record. I eagerly took the deal because I'd much rather tap into my savings to buy eight-tracks for my new stereo or the latest eyeshadow shade. I knew I needed help. (I was wild, not stupid.) Somewhere, in some far corner of my mind, a voice whispered that I shouldn't be doing all these bad things—hinted I was destined for something more—but I couldn't resist doing them anyway.

The psych eval diagnosed me with a conduct disorder. One of the referrals was to Briarpatch, an agency that intervened with troubled teens. Laura was my assigned case worker. Her skin was practically luminescent, her words laced with kindness, and her acceptance of anything I wanted to talk about unwavering.

I could count on her to be in her office week after week, listening to me rapt, as if what I was going through was essential and my processing of it valuable, interesting even. It felt awkward at first, being listened to so intently. Laura understood everything I shared, a perpetual source of validation, saying things like, 'You're very self-aware' and 'That's a pretty normal emotion for that situation.'

Her warmth enveloped me, in stark contrast to the criticism and dismissal I received at home. My guard lowered a little more each session. Things made more sense in her office. I left less angry than I came.

Finally, I had someone I could confide in, re-evaluate my decisions with, and form a more solid sense of myself. I didn't feel like such a weirdo after talking to Laura. I felt a lot less alone and eventually safe. So safe, I told her things I swore I'd never tell anyone—like how my Uncle Monte tickled me until I peed my pants.

"He can be up and on me before there's time to even *think* about running. Not that I could outrun him." His long arms and legs had me trapped in a cage that I writhed in the center of. His fingers were fast and strong, and the tickles hurt. "It's hard not to laugh, but I also scream for him to stop. I scream for someone, *anyone*, to do something—but no one ever does. They just say I'm overreacting. My family always says that whenever I'm upset. But it doesn't feel like overreacting to me. 'Stop being a baby,' Monte says when he finally releases me."

Then I'd flee upstairs, ashamed, to my grandparents' bathroom—the world blurred by the tears I tried to hold back—peel off my sour-smelling underwear and stuff it in the back of a closet. Eventually I'd come back down, wrapped in a blanket to hide the wet spot, humiliated and mumbling something about being cold.

Laura's face fell, confirming what I suspected. It wasn't okay. Not normal. "How does this make you feel?"

"Alone. Preyed upon. . . trapped. I feel betrayed by my relatives who are bigger, older, and able to defend me, but don't. They laugh like it's entertainment to them."

I couldn't understand why he didn't listen to me when I said stop, why no one took my cries for help seriously. Laura didn't understand either. That gave me a bit of relief. She didn't treat me any differently after I told her, giving me even more relief.

## GUT INSTINCTS

Laura ran a weekly group for teen girls, called Choices. Every Tuesday night, we gathered in Briarpatch's big old house on a hill—baking, crafting, watching movies, then spilling out onto the porch to talk about our broken homes and how we'd been broken in the process. The safety to speak freely without judgment or retribution was dizzying. Cathartic. Every week, I swept out from the dark corners of my mind and re-examined in the light.

My sense of belonging amplified every time I heard a girl say she missed her dad. Some didn't even know who their dad was. We entertained alternatives to handle our explosive emotions, ones that wouldn't solicit the attention of the police and land us back in court. Some of us sat on steps; others leaned against railings; all of us gathered there to get through this thing called life.

*None* of us really trusted anyone.

Honest conversations were missing from all our homes. So were people like Laura. She shrugged off the mistakes we made—even when the smoke alarm pierced the gray air because one of us forgot to set the oven timer. I'd never experienced anything like it.

I loved to help Mom bake, but if I spilled while measuring the vanilla or accidentally tipped the beaters, splattering cookie dough onto the wall, Mom would take over, elbowing me out and shooing me to the kitchen table to wait for a beater to lick.

Tuesday nights were my break from the pressure to perform, and I relished it. Making a mess or mistake was just part of the process. The radical acceptance was incredibly relaxing. Baking became *fun*. Week by week, I shed the costumes: tough girl, bad girl, trying-to-gain-approval-but-really-don't-give-a-fuck girl.

## JENNIFER JUNIPER

In that big old house, chaos wasn't punished. Messes weren't moral failures. They were just part of the process. Bit by bit, I shone outside the shadow of my family. My self-esteem rose from its bargain basement level, where I kept my prices so low that others had to buy. I could almost measure it from week to week, in mental notches, like one would a child's height on a door frame from year to year. (Not on any of my door frames, but I'd seen it on TV.)

I never wanted to get out of Laura's car, didn't want that golden sense of belonging to end. I felt safe inside the Tuesday night bubble of the Choices group. A bubble I tried to maintain and preserve, but something at home always popped it.

At the end of the twelve-week program, I had become a new version of myself: tamer and worthy of love and support. I made better decisions. . . for a while. In a radical departure from the norm, I gave my heart to a soft-spoken guy with quiet strength and tender eyes that didn't look away. Kevin gently extended all the support I longed for.

He offered his car for my driver's test—took it to a mechanic first, just to make sure everything worked. "Don't want you docked any points," he'd said.

I impressed the examiner, who passed me and said with flare, "You can parallel park my car anytime!"

Perched on the roof outside his bedroom window, Kevin broached the topic of sex with sweetness and respect. I'd never talked about it before. Just got swept away—wild and wordless—in the throes of raging hormones.

On our ride home from Planned Parenthood, a little paper bag of protection balancing and crinkling between us, I did mental gymnastics to figure out the best time of day to be consistent. I was terrified of getting pregnant. I recommitted to a decision made in health class my senior year, when I read that people tend to parent the way they'd been parented—a chance I couldn't take. (I'd even asked the doctor about getting my tubes tied. He patted my knee, told me I was young and would change my mind. But I wouldn't. I *couldn't.*)

Kevin confessed to being worried when the appointment went longer than planned, "I called the clinic to make sure you were alright."

The warmth of this concern wrapped around me. I had a boyfriend who cared enough to stand with me in the significant moments and steady my rites of passage. I basked in the rays of his caring companionship—until it started to burn.

Self-doubt whispered to me late at night, stared back from the mirror in the morning. *He's too good for you. You're out of your league.* The ease of us became uncomfortable. I was in a foreign country and I didn't speak the language. I got nervous—afraid of being exposed for the dark and twisted mess I was.

I wanted love, but love terrified me more than the prospect of abandonment. Kevin saw me, and that felt more dangerous than being invisible. *It's just a matter of time before he finds someone better.*

I did the only thing I could do—break up with him before he broke up with me.

I didn't even have the courage to do that. I did something worse—cheated on him with a guy who was cooler, edgier, and who ended up doing me dirty the same way. Relationship failures stacked themselves on top of the original sin I committed with Todd, my high school sweetheart. I kept doing rotten things and kept being a person I didn't like. The weight of that mix of memories pulled me further down in my second-hand sofa.

As I teetered on the edge of a whole new career direction, I had one final thought before fully committing to my new major. *I don't know if I'll make much money—Laura's car was pretty old—but it'll probably help me with my own fucked-upness.*

---

**Core Theme / Emotional Wound:** *Self-worth, betrayal, and the ache for belonging.* The journey from being a misfit to making empowered choices—and learning the cost of betraying yourself for acceptance.

**Gut Instincts Healing Method Stage:** *Follow.* Taking steps based on intuition and healing values, even if you're not sure where they lead yet.

**Old Survival Pattern:** *Seeking belonging* through external validation; *shapeshifting* to be chosen rather than choosing oneself.

**Reflection:**
Laura's warmth gave me a glimpse of what support could look like. Kevin's steady care offered a glimpse into a healthy partnership. But I wasn't ready to receive either. I didn't trust that I deserved them. So I sabotaged.

That part still stings—the pattern of burning down what I sincerely wanted because it felt too good, too foreign, too safe. I kept choosing chaos over calm because chaos felt like home.

But even in those choices, I was inching toward clarity. Each misstep was data. Each heartbreak cracked something open. I didn't know how to love myself yet, but I was learning what love wasn't.

## GUT INSTINCTS

The turning point didn't look heroic. It looked like serving Diet Coke to someone everyone else ignored. It looked like saying "yes" to a catalog that nudged something awake in me. My life didn't pivot overnight. But a quiet kind of compass was beginning to stir. And every time I followed that faint signal, I reclaimed a piece of myself.

Maybe that's what it means to "go your own way." Not in one grand declaration, but in thousands of small, defiant steps back to yourself.

**Reader Reflection:**

1. **Witness Your Self-Sabotage Without Shame:** Reflect on a time you pushed away something good—then trace the *why*. Was it fear? Unworthiness? A trauma echo? What did you learn from that experience? How do you work through fears of vulnerability or not being "enough"?
2. **Belonging and Healing:** The Choices group as a "bubble" of safety and support. Where do you feel most safe and accepted? How can you create more of these spaces in your life?
3. **Dreams vs. Expectations:** Have you ever felt pressured to follow someone else's idea of success? What steps did you take—or could you take—to prioritize your dreams over others' expectations?
4. **Embody the "Yes."** Choose one area of life where you feel stuck. Pause. Listen. What's the next intuitive "yes" that scares you a little—but also lights something up? Take one step in that direction.

JENNIFER JUNIPER

## Affirmation:

*I trust the path I'm on.
I am worthy of care that doesn't hurt and love that stays.*

Scan the Code Below to View the Video for Chapter 11:
Or go to: https://youtu.be/T8DDvL1fqdw

# Chapter 12

# Breaking Point

**When Your Inner Wisdom Demands to Be Heard**
When keeping it together falls apart,
there's beauty in the breakdown.

*Even the darkest night will end, and the sun will rise.*
~Victor Hugo

After a year of school, I switched to a secretarial position with steady money and benefits. The door to the plastics plant opened right by my desk. The second shift supervisor—*Josh*, according to the embroidered name patch on his navy-blue mechanic's uniform—came through often, accompanied by two distinct scents: the smell of burnt plastic and an air of easygoingness. Even with a machine's alarm clanging behind him, a smile flattened out his mustache, and his gait stayed relaxed.

He always had a corny joke locked and loaded, one that made his shoulders bounce when he delivered the punch line. I marveled at such evenness, as one would at an exotic animal. I'd be stressing over *another* typo on a purchase order—rifling through my desk for White-Out (and pink-out and yellow-out because the form was in triplicate)—and he'd cut right through my tension with a wink, a joke, a story, releasing the pressure like opening a can.

Casual exchanges in passing extended into his lingering at my desk. Years of grease embedded into the lifelines and love lines of his palms where soap couldn't reach, stimulating my imagination. *Looks like he's good with his hands.*

Lingering turned to leaning his dusty, navy-blue backside against a corner of my desk as he asked about my weekend, how I did on that test I was worried about, or made faces in the direction of my supervisor's cubicle while I rolled my eyes. No matter how upset or stressed I felt, he could always make me laugh.

"What's your extension?" He asked so he could call me from the plant with a part number.

"Twenty-one."

That answer brought him from leaning on my desk to leaning in a little closer. His big eyes turned flirtatious; his perma-smile went one-sided in a smirk. "Sooo, you're 21?"

"Yep!" I was surprised how naturally lying still came to me. I squashed my guilt by reasoning that, technically, it was true (even though I knew he was fishing for my age to see if I could get into bars). At 5'10", I'd been getting into bars since I was seventeen, so I didn't see the risk in faking it until I made it to twenty-one in a year.

Josh calmed things down for me, and I sure livened them up for him. He took his break when I had a gap between classes. We'd squeeze in a drive-thru dinner date—ten minutes of quickly stuffing our faces, followed by ten minutes of feverish backseat make-outs. I'd climb over the console and onto his lap, knee slipping on a Filet-o-Fish wrapper, using his erection as a pressure valve.

My whole body tingled during those little erotic vacations from my nonstop hustle of work, school, and top performance.

## GUT INSTINCTS

I felt powerful, making him want me. I went to my next class flushed and refreshed, convinced I had him—and life—by the balls.

I kept secrets even from myself. Both my inner and outer poker face stayed intact while a broken-glass blizzard swirled just beneath the surface of my skin. I could surf those waves of pain and chat about test scores or make weekend plans, all the while giving nothing away.

Disconnected as doll parts.

I'd pop them back together after it passed to the tune of delusion's greatest hits: It's Not That Bad and That'll Probably Be the Last Time. Secrets may have started as a foreign language, but they'd become my native tongue. My well-crafted life looked fine from the outside. But underneath? A body begging for help, and a mind sealing every crack with duct tape made of denial and determination.

Josh never challenged my stories. He was a shrugger. A whatever-er. Simple, easy, steady. I anchored to him like driftwood. He was the Bugs Bunny to my Tasmanian Devil. As I spun in chaotic tornado after chaotic tornado, he remained calm, comical, unflappable.

Weekend visits to his family's permanent campsite were more than intermissions of fun in a seriously packed planner: they were portals into a normal family. We sat around the fire, soup cauldron balancing on a tripod to share with visitors, then moved to a picnic table and shook dice for Ship, Captain, Crew until late in the night. His family was welcoming, accepting, and supportive, with everyone accounted for. No drama. No surprises. If I couldn't be normal, at least I could be *with* normal.

We'd been together about a year when Josh announced he was transferring plants and buying his sister's and brother-in-law's trailer up north in the rural outskirts of the tiny town of Neshkoro, where we stayed when we visited. "I'm coming with you," I blurted—a reflex, not reason. It wasn't a decision. It was a lifeline. *Don't leave me...* echoed in the hollow of my chest.

I framed it as a change of scenery. It was more like culture shock. A tiny town of 700. A trailer seven miles outside of it. Starry skies instead of city lights. Silence where there once was a din.

The first snowstorm trapped me inside, and the sensation of being a caged wild animal emerged—pacing, cursing, clawing at the door. I missed all my classes that day and raged at Josh over the phone, blaming him like he'd dragged me here against my will.

I compressed my classes into a three-day schedule and forfeited any extracurriculars. I avoided walking past the dance studio that called to me, but I pretended not to hear. I'd started ballet when I was five—in junior high, advanced to a pointe ballerina in pink satin shoes two sizes too small.

Now, instead of twirling, I was trudging. A full course load, a long commute, back to working as a waitress, all in the shadow of a body screaming for relief. But I stayed the course. Pushed myself. Hard. My drive was ferocious. My denial airtight.

Until it wasn't.

Being on a sprawling four-year university campus added amenities that a small community college didn't offer, like a building with Student Health Services chiseled into its brick facade and ivy vines pointing up to it in invitation. When my three-month supply of birth control pills got low, I chose the easier route of strolling across campus over finding the local Planned Parenthood.

My pen danced around the answers on the Health History Intake Form. I held the clipboard while a very familiar

# GUT INSTINCTS

vice grip of pain held my waist in its clutches. The more I told myself it was nothing, the more my body begged to differ. The pain wasn't easing up, and my ability to fake it was starting to fail me, too. Probably because a few days ago, I'd barely made it to the toilet on time and the horror of almost shitting my pants—or worse, leaving a trail of it in the hallway of the Education Sciences building—hung over me.

The pen hovered over the empty box next to Stomach Problems; the intense pain raging through my bowels a veritable plea for an honest answer.

I skipped it.

Went to the easier questions—like on any test—Asthma, Headaches, Fainting. Nope. Nope. Nope. Although I'd often wished it were any other part of my body breaking down. *Anything*, save for my girl parts, would be less embarrassing and a welcome trade for the mortifying discussion of poop and gas. I bargained with my bowels: if the pain passed before I finished the form, I'd leave the Stomach box blank.

Fierce independence was the superglue holding my full life and fragile tummy in place, sustained by the compulsion to keep it together while I was quietly falling apart. I wasn't quite ready for the hell sure to break loose if I let go of my control. Beneath the terror of telling where it hurt and for how long, lurked another layer with the three words I couldn't say: I need help.

The memory of my most embarrassing moment decided to plead its case. A few weeks prior, a sudden, burning urgency overtook me while driving to school.

I did the only thing I could do: pushed the pedal to the metal, trying to outrun the runs. Thankfully, the officer was the compassionate type and offered me an escort to the nearest gas station instead of issuing a ticket. I made it there with only dirty underwear, which I considered a blessing.

*I can get through the day without underwear.*

But it definitely put a dent in my denial. *What if there's a next time? What if I'm not that lucky?*

I sighed in defeat. Unclipping and flipping the form, I checked the Stomach Problems box, a reluctant witness testifying to my troubles. It felt like tearing down a brick from the wall I'd spent years building to protect myself. I handed it to the receptionist with my head lowered in shame, then sat in defeat as I waited.

"Jennifer. . .?" The nurse's voice snapped me back to the present.

---

**Core Theme / Emotional Wound:** *Denial as self-preservation.* Hiding illness out of fear and shame.

**Gut Instincts Healing Method Stage:** *Face* — The truth of what isn't working, even when it threatens the identity we've constructed around being capable, self-sufficient, and fine.

**Old Survival Pattern:** *Over-functioning as avoidance.* Denying needs to maintain the illusion of control and competence.

**Reflection:**
The most dangerous pain isn't always the sharpest—it's the one we learn to live with. The slow-burn symptoms that we normalize.

The warning signs we override. I didn't know it then, but every "I'm fine" was a brick in the wall between me and healing. I thought I was handling everything, but what I was really doing was white-knuckling life. Gaslighting myself while quietly preparing for worst-case scenarios.

# GUT INSTINCTS

Looking back, I can see how high-functioning denial gave me a false sense of control. But the cost was steep. I wasn't just running from pain—I was running from myself. The shame of needing too much, of being too messy, too complicated, too sick kept me silent. I know now that the body breaks down not to betray us, but to finally make us listen.

At some point, we all reach a point where the old strategies stop working. When I finally checked the box for Stomach Problems, it felt like a betrayal. But it was the beginning of truth-telling. Our bodies don't lie. They hold every secret we are too scared to say aloud. Mine had started to speak louder than I could ignore. Maybe yours is too.

**Reader Reflection:**

1. **Facing Denial:** Is there an area of your life where you might be downplaying or ignoring a problem? What's one small, honest step you can take today to acknowledge it?
2. **Coping Mechanisms:** Consider the ways you manage stress or pain. Are these strategies helping you heal, or are they keeping you stuck?
3. **Balancing Determination and Self-Care:** When you push yourself to achieve or "hold it together," do you also leave space for your body and emotions to rest? What would it look like to extend the same grace to yourself that you give to others?
4. **Seeking Help:** Why is asking for help often so difficult? If you could ask for support without judgment, what would you say and to whom? Where in your healing journey have you tried to be the "perfect patient"—

and what would it feel like to prioritize being your own fiercest advocate instead?
5. **Compartmentalizing vs. Integrating:** Are there parts of yourself or your life that you keep separate from others? What might shift if you allowed those parts to integrate into the whole?

## Affirmation:

*I am worthy of support in every season of my strength.*
*I choose to listen and be honest even when it's messy.*

Scan the Code Below to View the Video for Chapter 12:
Or go to: https://youtu.be/gZ2IdoAmDaQ

## Chapter 13

# Doctor!

**The Limits of Denial**
What happens when the "experts" don't have the answers?
Who do you trust then?

*It's not the load that breaks you down,
it's the way you carry it.*
~Lou Holz

I began cautiously painting the picture of my condition with the protection of a broad brush. "It feels like I have the flu." That was my safe, universally relatable response whenever the topic of my tummy troubles came up. It conveyed all the right symptoms: nausea, fatigue, loss of appetite, diarrhea, stomach cramps that folded me in half.

But I knew it wasn't that. *No flu lasts this long.*

The nurse held the thermometer up to the light. "No fever."

I told her my digestive system didn't seem to like food, flat-out rejecting it at times. "Kind of ironic, isn't it? Considering digestion is a major part of its job description?"

We laughed a little, and then she stopped and empathized. "Definitely not how it should work."

"Sometimes, it comes on so quickly with such force that I barely make it to the toilet in time. I'm sweaty and exhausted afterward."

The nice nurse scribbled something in my chart—fresh, new, and thin, the manila folder still crisp. She logged the first entry on an unsullied page titled NOTES.

"That sounds pretty rough. How long has this been going on?" Her warm tone inviting.

I sucked in a breath like I was doing the math, but I already knew. I held it in while I weighed the truth, entertaining a lie. Truth won by a hair, and I jumped into the deep end of honesty for a change. "About six years."

Her eyebrows shot up, and I scrambled to deflect her shock. "It was on and off. But lately, it's getting worse. I'm always scoping for a bathroom."

"You poor thing. It's good you came in." The stool squeaked as she turned from my chart to face me directly, her expression full of purpose. "I think we'd better have a doctor look at you."

Her words had no place to land in me. A frantic inner worrying whipped up like a storm, clouds of doubt and fear crowded my mind. I tried to keep it together as she patted my knee and assured, "It's better to know what we're dealing with."

*Depends on what we're dealing with.*

I flipped through a magazine while I waited, feigning nonchalance. But the stories were a blur, drowned out by a different kind of belly rumble—that of a scared little girl. *What will the doctor do to us? We shouldn't have said anything!*

My throat seized with fear and regret. I wished I could roll my words back onto my tongue and swallow them. But words heard become shared property, and the nurse was already spreading them further. My misgivings had lost the power of containment.

The doctor's white hair matched his white coat—his gentle eyes and kind smile conveyed concern, not horror. His very presence lowered my wariness to DEFCON 3. I looked down at my bloated belly, always giving me away, distended to pregnancy proportions—another irony, given this was an appointment to prevent such a thing. My hands rested on it as I talked, comforting it. Guarding it.

"It's like whatever I'm digesting hits a bottleneck and starts gurgling all down the line as if to say: 'Narrow passageway, we'll have to go through single file!' The backing up bloats me even more, and sharp pain makes the whole process unbearable. Heartburn rises in my chest. I burp up whatever I last ate. I worry I'll throw it up."

The doctor didn't seem disgusted by any of it (but I sure was). "How many bowel movements do you typically have in a day?"

"Seven. Ten. I can have three before lunch. Sometimes, I'll turn around and go right back into the bathroom after leaving it." I described the consistency, like brown liquid shooting from a fire hose, and the logistics of planning my life around bathroom locations. God forbid it was a single-seater. Stalls were better for hiding and strategizing. The deep shame of being heard or smelled added a layer of torture to an already humiliating situation. I'd try my best to hold it until the other person flushed, or I'd flush mine, to cover the noise.

"Hmm... any constipation?" His look quizzical.

"I wish! That would be a welcome reprieve."

It felt more like a confession than an intake, and there was some relief in sharing my burden. The doctor didn't blame or admonish me for waiting so long to seek help. His nod was slow and steady as he alternated between listening and taking notes.

He shook his head at the right parts, deflating a little of my fear and nurturing a fledgling trust.

But Brenda's story of waking up mid-colonoscopy lurked in the corner of my mind, cautioning me to tell enough to get help but not so much that he'd say, 'I think we should put a camera up your butt.'

The doctor suggested it might be a food allergy. "Why don't you keep a food diary for two weeks? Write down everything you eat, the amount and time, and any symptoms that follow. It should reveal the culprit."

At our next appointment, we pored over my diary like detectives searching for clues. No single food jumped out as the problem. No rhyme or reason to my misery. Still unpredictable.

We eliminated dairy. No change.

"Try leaving out wheat. No pasta or bread products."

That one was tough, but it didn't make a difference anyway. At each visit he floated a theory, and in every follow-up I debunked it. Hope was born anew only to be dashed by the evidence scribbled across my pages. No single food made it worse, and no elimination made it better.

It was like failing a class I never signed up for.

The kind yet frustrated doctor sighed as my junior year neared its end. "I'm afraid we've exhausted my expertise. I don't know what you have, but it's serious. You need to see a specialist. Let them run some tests."

It was the gentlest of breakups. Sincere compassion softened the blow before the brick of reality sank into my gut. I had no health insurance.

He suggested getting on my mom's policy, but he didn't know my mother. She and I weren't speaking, which was an improvement. To get her help would mean swallowing my pride and paying a steep emotional price.

*But am I not already paying dearly?*

Admitting my illness to a doctor had changed something. I couldn't stuff it back into a hidden compartment and keep pretending. The truth was glaring—we'd spent a semester investigating and I was no closer to a culprit, adding fear to frustration.

Interventions: 8 Improvements: 0

I was on borrowed time, and I knew it.

---

**Theme / Emotional Wound:** Asking for help equals weakness. Vulnerability leads to abandonment.

**Old Survival Pattern:** *Minimizing, avoiding, and delaying help out of fear* of what you'll find—or what it will cost to be taken seriously.

**Gut Instincts Healing Method Stage:** *Face*—The reality of illness, the emotional toll of being dismissed, and the fear of being seen as "too much."

**Reflection:**
For years, I was fluent in denial. But this chapter marks the point where that language starts to falter. Saying the symptoms out loud—writing them in a food diary, even—was a radical act of truth-telling for someone raised to keep everything quiet and neat. The nurse's empathy, the doctor's patience, they softened the armor. But what hit hardest was the shift inside me: I couldn't unknow what I'd said. And I couldn't go back to pretending it was all in my head.

Maybe you've been there—chronic symptoms you downplay, appointments you postpone, questions you avoid asking because you're afraid of the answers. And beneath all that? A deep craving: to be taken seriously, to be believed, to be helped.

**Reader Reflection:**

1. **Speaking Our Truth.** When was the last time you sought professional help for your difficult situation? Reflect on the moment you reached out—what was going through your mind? What fears or doubts held you back? How did you feel after you spoke your truth?
2. **Coming Out of the Dark.** What role does denial play in your journey? Are there aspects of your health or your life that you've been avoiding or minimizing? What would it look like to confront those things, even if it's just a small first step?
3. **Vulnerability Grants Access, not Abandonment.** How do you feel about the medical system and other helping professions? Think about your experiences with doctors and support providers. Do you feel heard and understood? Have you ever had an experience where you felt truly seen?
4. **Understanding Your Body's Love Language.** What does it mean to trust yourself? Trust is a major theme in your healing journey. How can you begin to rebuild trust in your body, especially when it feels like it's betraying you? How do you balance others' advice with your own intuition?

GUT INSTINCTS

## Affirmation:

*My breakdown is sacred.*
*My truth is rising.*

Scan the Code Below to View the Video for Chapter 13:
Or go to: https://youtu.be/6QwUjlY5Bxc

## Chapter 14

# I Need A Hero

### Some Battles Can't Be Fought Alone
When hope and desperation collide.

*Trauma creates change you don't choose.*
*Healing is about creating change you choose.*
*~Michele Rosenthal*

I crossed campus towards the parking lot. The budding hopefulness of spring teased at my senses as the weight of what I had to do heaved against my ribcage. Safely alone in my car, the doctor's directive reverberated louder, bouncing off the doors and windows as well as the walls of my skull.

*I don't know what you have, but it's serious. You need to see a specialist. Let them run some tests.*

I pulled my jacket around me, as if a few inches of fabric could protect me from the memory clawing at the locked door I didn't open unless I had to—and even then, only with gloves on.

The last time Mom and I spoke was shortly after I moved out. I called from the floor of my apartment, curled up and feeling vacuumed out. My brain swirled with confusion, head heavy with regret. What happened the night before played endlessly on a videotape I couldn't eject, each repetition scraping away another layer of trust in myself.

I'd met him at a party—a friend of a friend. He was good looking and funny, interesting and flattering. I was a little drunk and very lonely. When his hot breath whispered in my ear, "Let's get outta here," my heart leapt at the idea of being chosen and the chance to be alone with him.

I nodded into his musky cheek.

I declined a drink but said yes to smoking a joint on his couch. Our laughter built with each puff and pass, tumbling us into each other. We started kissing. But when he began moving too fast, I blocked him.

At least I tried to.

He didn't listen. And he wouldn't take me home. My heart gasped in dread as I realized how far I was from safety and how stupid I'd been to trust him.

Afterward, I stood under a scalding shower, scrubbing at a dirtiness that the soap and water couldn't reach. Shame's heavy weight pressed down on me, its accusing voice loud and relentless. Desperate for answers, I dialed my mom, the cop. Surely she'd know what to do.

"What were you thinking, getting in a car with someone you don't know?" Her stern voice stabbed at me through the receiver.

A regret flitted across my mind from when I was around sixteen. Perhaps I should have said something after the night her drunk boyfriend came over, knowing full well she was at work, and making some excuse to come in. He hit on me, cornering me between the fridge and the kitchen wall. Ignoring my protests, he leaned in for a kiss. With all the ferocity in my being, I pushed him away and ran to my room.

For days, I tried to decide whether telling Mom would soften things between us or make them more jagged—so I said nothing.

## GUT INSTINCTS

Lying there on the floor, a few years later and feeling even more icky, I fantasized that telling would've improved our current interaction. But maybe it would've messed me up even further if she blamed me for it.

Shame surged, choking back my words. I ached for a maternal rally cry against the asshole who took my body without my permission—for the comfort of, 'Come home.' Instead, I shrank further under shame's weight, just like the night before under a stranger's body.

But the doctor's 'It's serious' plea to seek help scared me enough to reconnect with a mother I fought to keep safe distance from.

"Why do you need insurance?" she asked in her familiar, terse tone.

Pangs of guilt pierced my heart. I swallowed my frustration and toed the line between pleasing her and asking for what I needed. "Just in case something happens," my voice shrugged.

"Why? What's wrong? Is there something you're not telling me?"

Her voice took on its typical interrogative tone. I felt more on trial than on a call for help. My protective shields shot up. My stomach clenched, bracing me once again. It wasn't just paperwork. It was trying—one last time—to ask for care from someone I'd already stopped counting on. And still, I had to ask.

Still, I hoped.

"No. . . nothing's wrong," I stammered, riding that familiar line between giving enough but not so much that it could be used against me. "I just thought, you know, maybe get a physical."

I kept waiting for someone to swoop in, offer protection, or at least answers. But heroes didn't come for me. I was starting to understand that I had to become my own—even with cracked armor and a shaky sword.

Mom sighed her oh-so-familiar sigh of reluctant acquiescence. "Fine."

It wasn't a kidney—it was a line in an insurance policy with the premium covered by her job at the Sheriff's Department. Every student I knew was on their parents' policy.

Our conversation snapped me back to countless band concerts spent poised on the school's stage, scanning the audience for my habitually late mom. I'd pressed my sweaty fingers against the cool clarinet keys, heart leaping with every shift in the crowd, hoping for once she'd be there before the lights dimmed.

Eventually she'd appear, rushing into the stands between songs, her tardiness as predictable as my yearning.

---

**Theme / Emotional Wound:** *Betrayal + Abandonment.* The people who were supposed to protect you (your mother, the system, even your own instincts) didn't. And in the wreckage, you realized: no one's coming. You'll have to save yourself.

**Old Survival Pattern:** *Hyper-independence / Suppressed needs.* Don't ask for help, don't show weakness, handle everything alone. Stay small, quiet, ashamed. And it's costing you your health, happiness, and wholeness.

**Gut Instincts Healing Method Stage:** *Feel + Face.* This chapter lives in the tender, essential territory of feeling the old pain and facing the truth about what happened—without numbing, rationalizing, or shaming it away.

## Reflection:

Years later, I'd learn about 'the effects of being raised in an oversexualized environment.' Look at how growing up with Playboy magazine's lying around the house helped form Prince's style. And how mine got affected by a guy Mom wanted to marry, but we wouldn't see for weeks or months at a time. I'd hear his return, in the night, in loud moans and the knocking of her headboard against the wall just on the other side of mine.

It's hard enough to develop a solid sexual identity and healthy expression of it, but when adult extracurriculars bleed into your budding development, a True North becomes even more elusive. My compass would spin in that department for decades.

I'd been waiting for someone to rescue me—from pain, from shame, from myself. But maybe healing isn't about waiting for a hero. Perhaps it's about becoming the one you need. Have you ever reached out for help and gotten shut down, judged, dismissed, or ignored? Maybe it taught you not to ask again. Perhaps, like me, you began to believe you had to do it all alone. But healing doesn't happen in isolation. And your pain doesn't mean you're weak—it means you're human.

## Reader Reflection:

1. **Unmet Needs and Lost Protectors:** Who did I need to protect me that didn't—or couldn't? Who did I need most when I was hurting, and what did they not give me?
2. **Silencing and Self-Protection:** When have I shut down instead of speaking up or asking for what I need? What moments taught me that it was safer to stay silent?

3. **Redefining Strength and Vulnerability:** What's one belief I hold about needing help or being vulnerable? Do I equate "strong" with "silent"? Where did I learn that—and is it serving me now?

## Affirmation:

*I am the one I've been waiting for.
I carry the strength I once searched for in others.*

Scan the Code Below to View the Video for Chapter 14:
Or go to: https://youtu.be/SY6cfgLRcwo

## Chapter 15

# Help!

### The Fear of Knowing
When you're ready but they're not.

*Speak your truth, even if your voice shakes.*
~Maggie Kuhn

The parchment-papered table crinkled and stuck on the back of my naked thighs while I waited, reminding me of plucking pastries sticking to the lining of the tray at my grandma's bakery. My anxiety needed a distraction, so I entertained myself wondering which kind of pastry I was. A donut or more of the croissant type? Cream puff? Fragile as the phyllo of an apple turnover, ready to crumble at first bite?

I landed on cinnamon roll—tightly wound, tougher on the outside, gooey at the center with a bit of spice.

My legs dangled off the edge, swinging beneath the impossible-to-tie hospital gown. The overhead fluorescents highlighted their hairy stubble, triggering horror. *I should've shaved my legs!*

A different inner voice chimed in with quiet assurance. *He won't be looking at our legs.* It sounded like me, but upgraded—stronger, calmer, wiser.

My scared and worried voice mumbled back. "I wish he were looking at our legs."

The privacy of my bowel functions going public, spilling out of its compartment, left me exposed and without my typical tight grip on things. I felt faulty, like there wasn't just something wrong with me, but something *wrong with me*.

It stemmed from years of the ingrained message, 'if you can't figure it out, it's because you haven't tried hard enough.'

If you can't make Kraft Macaroni-n-Cheese properly—evidenced by my younger sister Lisa pouring neon orange liquid from her spoon while singing the Chunky Soup jingle: 'it's the soup that eats like a meal,'—it's *you*, not that you're too young.

A soft knock broke my reverie, snapping me back with a sharp inhale and pounding pulse. I braced for impact, reminiscent of all the times I'd been caught at something.

Left alone with my thoughts, the size of the exam room and my stomach problems had switched places, until they loomed large as a zeppelin. The doctor didn't so much enter the room as squeeze into it.

Doctor Number Two was younger than College Doc and without the gray hair I'd found so comforting—or maybe it's the bond formed with someone in my corner as I shadowboxed my symptoms.

"Soo," he said, more to the open file he held than to me. "You're having stomachaches."

I laid back on the table, exposing my shredded digestive system to pushing and probing, and rolled my eyes at how severely he'd understated my condition. Starting over again with someone else layered another level of vulnerability. I focused on finding designs in the dots of the drop ceiling and tried not to think about what new things this new guy might want to do to me.

## GUT INSTINCTS

At the same time, a small but vital inner voice whispered, *Help me*. Maybe that whisper was enough. In order to quell some of my immobilizing anxiety, I'd locked Brenda's scary story away, but I could still hear its muffled sounds of warning.

"Does this hurt?" Doc #2 asked, pressing exactly where it hurt.

"Uh-huh."

"How about over here?"

I winced and nodded.

"And here?"

I wanted to scream, IT ALL HURTS! Save him the trouble and me the torture. *That's why I'm here, for Chrissakes.* Instead, I pressed my lips tightly together and mumbled another "Mmm–hmmm," like a good patient.

"How long have you felt this way?" He gave me a hand sitting up.

It seemed like forever.

I tried to remember when my digestive system actually enjoyed food—processing it easily, instead of spewing it out in rejection. I thought back to a time before I was pulling over, scrambling for—praying there were—old drive-thru napkins in the glove box, and darting into the bushes on the side of some back road.

I counted backward from my twenty-two-year-old self, starting her senior year in college, to the first time my body took me down as a high school junior, doubled over, head sweating on the dash of a Monte Carlo.

"About seven years." It sounded incredulous even to me. It made me sound tougher, or crazier, than I actually felt.

His exhale was audible. "That's a long time."

"I've been busy," I defended, sounding lame. Like attending to my health was a pile of laundry I hadn't gotten around to folding.

I wasn't just busy—I was terrified. But terror's easier to outrun when it's dressed up as productivity.

He felt under my jaw. "Your lymph nodes are pretty swollen." He asked if anyone in my family had stomach problems. They didn't. "Ever pass blood?" God, no—one thing to be grateful for.

We talked about the number of daily bowel movements and their appearance—usually around eight, as high as ten, always unformed and feeling like hot lava—the urgency and force with which they painfully poured out of me, leaving me exhausted and depleted, blotting my sweat with toilet paper and splashing my face with water before dragging my body back to class.

All the hiding and lying were getting exhausting, too, forcing me to find the courage to face it fully.

"We'll start with blood work and a stool sample." Doctor Cold & Clinical was back at his desk, writing orders.

I told him about the food diary I'd kept last semester and the investigative elimination diet that College Doc and I'd done. "That doctor thought I needed to see a specialist." The paper sticking to my thighs crinkled as I leaned his way, hoping he'd write me a referral instead.

"Mm-hm." His head stayed down.

I'd been suffering for years, but now I'd punched my ticket in the medical machine. Surely, that meant the ride to recovery had begun. *Let's get me better. Fix it. Fix **me**.* I told him about getting pulled over for speeding, afraid I wouldn't reach the bathroom in time.

"We'll start with this." Handing me his orders.

In a last-ditch effort to sway him, I played my biggest card. The best way I knew to describe the brutality my body was capable of. "Sometimes it feels like I'm digesting razor blades."

His turn to wince. "That sounds painful."

*Surely, he'll advance me now.*

"We'll see what the test results show. Make a follow-up appointment with me in two weeks." He rose from his stool, signaling the end of the conversation.

They took fifteen vials of blood from me—every one, hard-won. The needle jabbed, and my veins would bob and weave. The tube would start to fill, then stop, making the phlebotomist's forehead crinkle. "Sorry, your veins keep collapsing." With alcohol and determination, she scrubbed a new spot.

I felt bad for both of us.

I'd look away, then peek back as she popped one tube off and clicked another on. I wondered how much blood a person could lose. Then I wondered what they would all find. And with fifteen vials, each with a different colored top, how many things were they looking for?

As I reached for the elevator button, my stomach clenched—not from pain, but some vague awareness.

I hadn't contemplated much on what was wrong with me, being in denial and all. I was busy pursuing the best grades, closing in on graduation, and planning to parlay the part-time job in my field into a full-time one. I was so hungry to start my career, I could taste it—or maybe that was stomach acid. Either way, it burned inside me.

But the gauze around my elbow held my attention.

*I'm too young to have cancer.*

Too young for my body to betray me. Denial had been a bandage I kept slapping on a wound without cleaning it first. It held me together, but left scars underneath.

It meant mistaking motion for progress. Hustle for healing. And convincing myself that collapsing later was still better than breaking down now.

Later had arrived, demanding answers I wasn't sure I was ready to hear.

---

**Theme / Emotional Wound:** *Shame + Fear of exposure.* You've been hiding behind high performance and self-sufficiency for so long that asking for help feels like a threat. Admitting something's wrong isn't just inconvenient—it feels like admitting *you* are wrong.

**Old Survival Pattern:** *Perfectionism + Denial as Control.* If you stay busy, you don't have to feel how bad it's gotten. If you play the good patient, maybe you won't have to confront what's really going on. You keep everything moving so you don't have to stop and unravel.

**Gut Instincts Healing Method Stage:** *Face + Feel.* This is the chapter where you can't "push through" anymore. The symptoms are louder than your stories, and the pain becomes the truth-teller. You begin to face your body's reality—and let yourself feel the fear, fatigue, and grief underneath it all.

**Reflection:**
We all have our versions of the parchment paper—those sterile moments when we finally stop pretending everything is okay. Maybe for you, it wasn't a doctor's office, but a diagnosis, a panic attack, a night you couldn't keep going. That's not failure. That's the beginning. The body never betrays—it only tells the truth you've been trying to outrun.

**Reader Reflection:**

1. **Self-Advocacy:** Have you ever hesitated to ask for help, even when you knew you needed it? What held you back, and how did you eventually find the courage to speak up?
2. **Navigating Uncertainty:** How do you manage fear or anxiety when facing the unknown, especially regarding your health?
3. **Trusting Yourself:** What role does intuition play in your decision-making, especially when others hold power over outcomes that affect you?
4. **Denial:** Have you ever ignored a problem because facing it felt overwhelming? What did it take for you to acknowledge it?

    How has denial served you in difficult times? When did it stop working for you? What small step could you take today toward facing something you've been avoiding?

## Affirmation:

*I am worthy of care, even when I'm a mess.*
*I deserve to be taken seriously.*
*My truth is worthy of attention and care.*

JENNIFER JUNIPER

Scan the Code Below to View the Video for Chapter 15:
Or go to: https://youtu.be/hr8MnwN_cQg

---

By the end of Part 2, you'll shift from resistance to receptivity, learn to interpret your experiences as information, not attacks.

---

Part Three

# Reclamation

## Stepping Into Full Healing & Freedom

*True liberation is not just about fixing what's not working —it's about reclaiming your life.*

## Chapter 16

# Don't Stop Believin'

**The Power of Decision**
Healing starts with choosing to believe it.
Others give opinions, but only you decide what's possible.

*When we are no longer able to change a situation,
we are challenged to change ourselves.*
~Viktor E. Frankl

There's just never a good day to poop in a cup. The empty container sat waiting on my bathroom counter, and I waited for a specimen of excellence to put in it. A diagnostic test was still a test after all, and tests were something to ace. (As if the will to make the brown liquid form into some kind of standard shape was enough. If that were true, I'd have willed it already. Long ago.)

We were in a standoff, the cup and I, at the *Not* Okay Corral.

But I couldn't advance to a specialist without it, so, after a few days, the cup won. I filled, sealed, and slid the mucousy liquid into a plastic bag plastered with biohazard warnings, then placed that inside a paper lunch bag and tied a plastic grocery bag around it. Poop smells pretty gross anyway, but poop from broken bowels has an alarmingly rancid stench.

# JENNIFER JUNIPER

*Should I enclose an air freshener? A clothespin? A note of apology?*

My sample sloshed shotgun until I moved it to the floor, fearing it would break out somehow and spill. Handing it over made me realize the only thing more horrific than seeing your soup-like poop (poop du jour?) captured in a cup is imagining someone else seeing it. And smelling it.

I walked into Quisling Clinic and smirked at the name swinging on a sign above me. *More like Quizling Clinic. I'll take Bizarre Bowel Functions for $1,000, Alex.* Opening the door, my sense of humor completely dissolved as that foreboding scent of sterility stung my nostrils. There was nothing funny about how my digestive system tortured me.

\*\*\*

I would never get the results of those tests. Would never see Doctor Cold & Clinical again.

Two days later, barely into the one-hour commute to campus, it started: stabbing pains, followed by the clutching cramps that bent me over and made me cross an arm over my belly, trying to soothe and calm it.

I crunched onto the shoulder to wait it out like a pop-up thunderstorm, resting my head on the race-car-themed steering wheel.

My yellow AMC Hornet was rusting through the flames painted on the quarter panels and burned oil. I blew the motor by ignoring the flashing red oil can for too long—a delay I often got away with. Until I didn't.

My body was also tired of being asked for more than it could give. I thought back to learning to drive stick in it. With no driver's ed instructor to save me when I stalled at an intersection, I just kept trying until I got it. That was how I did everything.

But no amount of grinding gears would get my belly going. I looked up at the on-ramp. *I don't think I'll be able to make it.*

There would be no waiting it out, breathing and denying until it passed, blinded by the hope that this time would be the last. I sighed my reluctant surrender, expelling years of delay. I'd been filing red flags into folders labeled 'Later.' My body screamed, and I chalked it up to a stress response, promising myself: *After this exam.*

*After this paper.*

*After I graduate.*

But 'later' never came.

I wasn't managing. I was flat-out denying. And learning denial doesn't protect you. It just delays the inevitable. My body, tired of being ignored, wasn't firing warning shots anymore. It was issuing ultimatums. The file cabinet had burst open—folders and papers flying wildly in the wind.

My hands shook against the stitched leather steering wheel, already bracing for the worst. Gravel again crunched under my tires—in applause or judgment, hard to tell—as I turned around and put the onramp in my rearview mirror.

No more running.

Luckily, I wasn't far from my close friend Lori's house—the one person who could see through the facade of strength I'd built so strong, for so long. Maybe because she had her own battle scars and a bad heart, giving her a window into my broken body. She knew when to push, when to soothe, and when to fight for the version of me I hadn't yet met.

I wished it was my heart that wasn't working, or a knee... pretty much *anything* else. Then it would be X-rays, MRIs, or wires connecting me to a machine. I could keep my underwear on for that at least, and be awake. My tests seemed like the most invasive possible: "Mind if we put a camera up your butt and have a look around?"

Lori opened the door, and Journey (she *only* listened to Journey) flowed out onto the stoop where I was sweating waterfalls, holding onto the doorframe for support.

I knew how bad it was by the look on her face.

"You look like a ghost!" She reached and pulled me in by my wrist, her other arm circling around my waist, guiding me tenderly to the couch. I laid down and melted into it. While she put a cold washcloth on my forehead, she put her foot down. "I've had enough of this. I can't watch it anymore. I'm calling the doctor."

She was a blue-eye-shadowed badass in her own right, AquaNet holding her bottle blonde waves in place. Lori had twenty years on me, often taking a more maternal tone in our friendship and telling me I should respect my elders in a tone that was only *half*-joking.

Too weak to fight, I knew she was right. It had gone on long enough. Too long. And my body was in on it. It could've given out anywhere. In class. On the highway. At work. But it chose to give out here, knowing it would be heard. Right down the road from the one person it knew it couldn't win an argument with.

If *Don't Stop Believin'* wasn't the song playing, it should have been.

Time stood still, or maybe it warped. Those swish-swoosh doors sealed me in and silenced the outside world. The homework in my backpack would have to wait; taking its place were different questions requiring more personal answers, setting me up for the kind of exams you can't study for. A bundle of anger, resignation, and fear, I balanced another clipboard on my thigh with pages and pages of words I barely read but signed anyway, granting permission for treatments without knowing what they are and implying trust in people not yet met.

*I'm sick of this shit. Just make me better.*

Being admitted to the hospital made me feel like my body was no longer solely mine. I was turning it over to medical science as a shared commodity. I was willing, but I was wary. I felt like I'd been running from it for so long, I was out of road. Caught. The IV my handcuffs. An IV that took seven tries to get in.

"I'm so sorry, your veins keep collapsing," the nurse said softly, her eyes darting to mine like she might break me with her worry. I could also hear what she *wasn't* saying: You've failed; can't be alone; can't sleep in your own bed. You need care that you can't provide.

I didn't want pity. I hated being seen as fragile. Fragile meant weak and vulnerable. Vulnerability signaled danger; the need to protect myself. Defend myself. Right or wrong, this was how the psychological dominoes fell in my head. It wasn't calculated or even conscious. There wasn't some off-switch I could flick, even if I had the self-awareness to look.

In my house, weakness was a liability. If you cried, you were 'making a scene.' I learned early: don't need. Don't break. Don't show it.

Some people feel relieved once they are admitted to the hospital, and a whole team springs into action, comprising those trained to help, diagnose, and treat a wide range of ailments. All questions will be answered. All problems will be solved. (One person I shared this with said, "I just love that feeling. It's so comforting to know that you're in the hands of professionals.")

## JENNIFER JUNIPER

That was not at all my experience. I guess when you have childhood memories chock full of doctors who can't fix you—the pink penicillin constantly in the fridge, tubes in my ears, my tonsils taken out, and yet ear infections continued to plague me—being in the hands of professionals isn't exactly comforting. Doctors and I had a long history together: them doing painful things in the name of helping me, and me, still sick, and having no choice but to go back for more.

Backed into a corner in a backless gown.

---

**Theme / Emotional Wound:** *Loss of control + Medical trauma.* You've crossed a threshold—your defenses are collapsing, and now you're forced to face the reality you've been trying to outrun. The wound is the loss of agency over your body, your safety, and how others see (or don't see) your pain.

**Old Survival Pattern:** *Over-functioning + Delay tactics.* I'll deal with it later. After this test. After this semester. After I earn rest. After I earn care. You've been postponing healing, hoping your performance could protect you.

**Gut Instincts Healing Method Stage:** *Feel → Face.* This is a breaking point—and a reckoning. You're forced to face what you've denied. But there is help. You don't have to do it alone

**Reflection:**
We all have our version of the "highway breakdown." The moment our body says, *I can't carry you like this anymore.* Maybe it wasn't pain in your gut, but panic in your chest, or fatigue so deep you couldn't get out of bed. Perhaps you were also handed a clipboard full of words you didn't read, just signed—and hoped someone, anyone, could fix you. It's

terrifying. But it's also sacred. Because that's the moment your old life ends, and something new begins.

Admittance to a hospital was my version of an alcoholic hitting rock bottom. But what if I didn't stay there? What if it wasn't the end of the road, but the beginning of something I'd never dared imagine—a life that didn't revolve around pain?

**Reader Reflection:**

1. **Facing the Breaking Point:** Have you ever ignored your personal check engine light, believing you could push it just a little farther? What happened when you finally reached your breaking point?
2. **Surrender as Strength:** What does surrender mean to me? What am I afraid will happen if I let go of control? How do you feel about the idea that surrendering can be a form of strength?
3. **The Power of Advocates:** Who is your "Lori"—the person who speaks up for you when you can't? How has their support shaped your journey?
4. **Trusting the Process:** Have you ever hesitated to seek help because of fear, distrust, or past experiences? What helped you push past that hesitation?
5. **Redefining Rock Bottom:** Rock bottom can become a solid foundation to rebuild. Can you identify a moment in your life that felt like rock bottom but ultimately became a turning point?

## Affirmation:

*My breaking point is the beginning of my breakthrough.
I am allowed to rest.
I am allowed to receive.
My decision to trust myself is the first,
and most powerful, step forward.*

Scan the Code Below to View the Video for Chapter 16:
Or go to: https://youtu.be/GtPQ5EmD0Z4

**Chapter 17**

# Landslide

### The Collapse Before the Clarity
When everything feels like it's falling apart,
sometimes it's clearing the way for something new.

*Sometimes, when you're in a dark place,
you think you've been buried,
but you've actually been planted.*
~Christine Caine

The hospital room was cold in a myriad of ways—temperature, construction, sterility. Cold tiles, metal beds, aluminum poles, white skritchy sheets, the IV fluid running cool into my veins. And that always flapping open, impossible to get on right, gown—with cold metal snaps.

I felt an internal cold, too. The isolation of being sick and broken and on display. A specimen, an anomaly, a freak of nature strangers whirring around me trying to decode me with intimate questions that were embarrassing to answer. A chronic condition make you feel all alone, even if someone else is in the room.

I had a private room at least, *that* isolation I was grateful for, with a window to watch a tree fill with fresh green leaves, coming back to life in the breeze. Spring meant second-semester midterms, but my mind focused on other exams. The ones the doctor was talking about.

Doctor #3, a gastroenterologist (finally!), burst on the scene like a man with a mission, his long stride, made the flap of his white lab coat splay open as he walked. He arrived at my bedside with a clipboard and confidence, swooshing his hair out of his eyes before he began.

"We're going to draw some blood, run some tests. I've scheduled an endoscopy and colonoscopy for tomorrow morning. It's a camera on the end of a tube, one going in through your mouth and the other in through your rectum. It allows me to see inside your entire digestive system. I'll take biopsies and check for any pre-cancerous cells. I'll remove any polyps I find. You'll do the prep tonight—a cleanse for better visibility."

"That should be easy. I doubt there's much in there." I attempted a smile.

A warm smile returned, saying he understood. "By this time tomorrow, we'll know exactly what's wrong with you."

I exhaled fully for the first time since I'd arrived. *He gets it. I've finally found someone who knows what we're dealing with.* His certainty brought relief and lowered the freak factor. *He's seen this before.* A tenuous bond formed between us. My guard lowered. The doctor was competent and compassionate (and cute!). I was in good hands. I could feel it.

After he left the room it all hit me, *hard*. Something in me broke open. I'd lost twenty-five pounds and hadn't even noticed. *What the hell!?* It wasn't just the overwhelm of my sick situation—it was everything I'd been holding back and all the things I didn't know how to deal with gushing out behind it.

I started to spin out.

I felt so helpless. So vulnerable. Not just because of the draft breezing up my backside. Because I was terrified of the fallout. I prided myself on having my shit together, needed to be seen in this light. Not because I was vain—more like a vampire.

Like the exposure would kill me.

The invasive nature of what he was proposing, the intensity of the prep, the guilt of my procrastination—it all started to swirl. The unconscious state I'd be in around people I'd only just met—my lack of control over any of it. I was losing what little grip I still had on the situation. *These people are strangers, and they're taking over.*

That was what I'd been afraid of every time in the ER roundabout—big things happening to me and me being powerless.

Powerless over a tummy refusing to let me push the pedal to the overachievement metal. It wouldn't be enough to graduate wearing a cap and gown—I had to have an honors cord. Driven by some deficit I couldn't reconcile.

All the time and energy spent running, resisting, covering up, and compensating was caving in. I cried tears I'd been carrying for years, and they spilled a mix of fear, shame, and surrender. The defenses I deployed to avoid the very place I was in were emptying out of me, and it was messy.

Snot and tears and sobs turned to wails of sheer terror, making my chest heave and hurt. The force of an emotional tsunami rocked my body on its own. I was a vessel caught in a storm I couldn't steer.

"That's it. Let it alllll out." Brenda cooed from her vinyl visitor recliner.

Suddenly, yet softly, an invisible blanket of protection and certainty wrapped around me. A hush fell over my churning mind, and I stopped crying mid-sob. Something had lifted my burden, shining away clouds and shrouds I'd been living under for the past seven years, vanishing my shame like magic.

The Presence was vast—too expansive to be contained by my circumstance—and it steadied the storm that had erupted inside me. I knew instantly that I could trust it. Its warmth in stark contrast to the cold of my room (and my reality). So powerful it sucked the sadness, fear, and suffering right out of me.

The whole thing was a little alarming, but mostly amazing. Odd, yet familiar. Heavy, but not oppressive, just demonstrating its breadth and strength. I melted into it.

It had to be God, but I didn't remember praying—although I often did, and in less dire circumstances. Conscious prayers that asked for concrete things, like *help me remember* when I sat down to a test, or a plea to avoid cops as I sped to make up time because I'd overslept. And I always prayed for the pain to stop—with my arms crossed and clutched around my middle instead of lacing my fingers together.

It was a wordless answer to a wordless prayer. Calm seeped deep into the center of me and dropped anchor.

Brenda was stunned at how abruptly I'd stopped crying. "What just happened?"

An encounter with the divine is hard to describe—it truly is 'a peace that surpasses all understanding.' "I'm not sure," I said softly. Humbled. "I think God might be here."

Everything looked the same, but I felt different. Freshly showered, but on the inside.

Like that time waiting for my dad and watching the leprechaun scene develop in the grass, I felt those big, invisible arms hold and carry me—comforting and strengthening me. As if the poster from my childhood bedroom door had come to life: *Lord, help me to remember that nothing's going to happen today that You and I can't handle together.*

Where was all that bad and fearsome, I am a jealous God stuff I'd heard from the pastor jumping up and down in the pulpit? It seemed to me that God was the essence of all the good things in life, distilled down and recreated without having to go anywhere or pay anything.

I hadn't even asked. Unless God took my freaking out and all the sobs and snot and as a request—which it totally was.

By the time my sister arrived with the items I'd requested, the mood in my hospital room had significantly improved. Smiles surfaced, along with a growing belief that I could handle whatever came next. Somehow, I trusted it would all be okay. Lisa announced her presence with a look of concern, a sigh of relief, and a triumphant "Finally!"

Absorbed by and consumed with propelling myself through life, I hadn't for one moment considered the effect my decisions had on others. I realized it then, in the look on her face. I watched her unpack the bag she'd brought and settle in, her movements reiterating her sentiment on the phone, 'I'll stay with you until it's done.'

It was about as party-mode as you can get with a gallon of laxative perched on your tray table. We rolled the backgammon dice, trying to pretend it was just another night in—until my belly began rumbling louder than the game board.

"Golytely?" she smirked. "More like *Goquickly*!" giving me my only chuckle of the night.

And so began the shuffle: backgammon, belly grumble, bathroom. With an IV pole in tow, toilet breaks became a new form of cardio. Before flushing, I'd ring the nurse, sure I'd achieved the "poop-until-it's-clear" directive. Each time the nurse would shake her head, rub my back, and pour another glass.

It was like swallowing the ocean.

When I finally got to where they wanted me to be, empty, I was raw. I climbed back into bed, no longer caring about my backside hanging out. My underwear, which I'd insisted on keeping as some sort of pièce de la résistance, was dirty and discarded. The one barrier I had, flimsy as it was, gone.

I drifted into sleep, wishing again for it to be any other part of my body breaking down instead.

'By this time tomorrow, we'll know exactly what you have.' I let it play on repeat as I drifted off to sleep.

Breakfast the next morning was a magic elixir of mist served through a mask over my nose and mouth. With every number I counted backward, my mind blurred further into euphoria. All my problems, my faults, struggles, all that I lacked, evaporated as I drifted off, weightless.

Before floating away completely, I moved the mask to the side, and groggily told the anesthesiologist hovering above me, "This makes that prep *totally* worth it."

He moved the mask back into place with a chuckle. "Yeah, I get that a lot."

Waking up back in my room, I strained to make out the fuzzy figure at my bedside table. *Hmmm. . . he's cute. . . kinda familiar. . . Oh! It's Doctor Cute and Confident!* Bent over a piece of paper showing the outline of a man and his digestive system—like he'd swiped a coloring sheet from the children's wing playroom—he held a black pen instead of crayons. He'd already drawn dashes down the throat and throughout the stomach. As I fought to emerge from the cloud of anesthesia and blinked to focus, he was heading into the colon.

"What are those?" I squeaked and squinted.

He glanced up. "You're awake." Then went back to drawing dashes throughout the maze of intestines. "Ulcers. You're full of 'em!"

# GUT INSTINCTS

**Theme / Emotional Wound:** *Powerlessness + Invisibility*
You've feared what would happen if you truly let go. That fear rooted itself in the need to be perfect, polished, and capable of handling anything. But you can't outrun it anymore. And in the breakdown, you're finally *seen*.

**Old Survival Pattern:** *Hypervigilance + Control Through Competence.* Coping by being on top of everything—grades, work, appearances. Push. Perform. Produce. Present. It's all a regulation mask. A survival strategy that turns into high-functioning. It's the "I'm fine" façade that protects you from the shame of being seen as weak, needy, or "too much."

**Gut Instincts Healing Method Stage:** *Face + Feel.* This is a layered transition. *Facing* reality. *Feeling* the grief, terror, shame. You learn that letting go is sometimes the most powerful thing you can do.

**Reflection:**
I don't recall Josh being there at all, which is weird. He was probably working, but still...

Sometimes the real healing starts when your body is empty, your pride is gone, and you're half-naked in a hospital gown playing backgammon with your sister. It begins when you let someone hold you—spiritually, emotionally, literally—and realize that needing help doesn't make you weak. It makes you human. Maybe even holy.

Remember the meaning of a cappella? *In the manner of the chapel. Just soul and resonance in pure form.* The sound is sacred *because* it's stripped down. Just like the threshold to healing. That moment when everything external is taken away, and all that's left is your truth echoing in the quiet. It's sacred in its own brutal way.

A note about God: to quote Dolly Parton, "You gotta believe in a Power greater than yourself." That's how you achieve the big things your little self can't. You get to define it. It can even be your higher Self. That inner compass that guides you when you're uncertain. The aspect of yourself that seems to know the way forward, even when your mind is confused.

**Reader Reflection:**

1. **The Power of Vulnerability.** Have you ever felt completely vulnerable or powerless in a situation? What helped you move forward and find peace?
2. **Divine Intervention.** Do you believe in moments of divine intervention or unexplainable calm? If so, how have these moments shaped your perspective on life?
3. **Loss and Renewal.** When have you experienced the catharsis of an emotional release? What did you learn about yourself through the process?
4. **Human Connection Amid Struggle.** Who are the "angels" in your life who show up when you need them the most? How do their actions inspire you?
5. **Releasing the Need to Be "Put Together".** Do I equate being "put together" with being lovable or safe? Where am I still trying to earn love or safety by appearing perfect?
6. **Finding Peace in Surrender.** Have you ever experienced a moment of surrender that felt like peace? What might soften in your life if you stopped fighting what is and started trusting what could be?

GUT INSTINCTS

## Affirmation:

*I reclaim the abandoned parts of myself.
I am becoming whole in the spaces
where I let myself be held.*

Scan the Code Below to View the Video for Chapter 17:
Or go to: https://youtu.be/Gqq96JTMG08

## Chapter 18

# You Learn

### Two Types of People
Some accept the prognosis. Others explore possibilities.

*Your body hears everything your mind says.*
~Naomi Judd

"The good news is, we know what you have. Crohn's disease characterized by ulcerations and inflammation throughout the digestive system."

"Never heard of it." While I floated in leftover anesthesia, my mind braced for the blow.

"It's an autoimmune disorder. Your body is attacking itself."

"Why would it do that?"

"We don't know. Either you have something in you that no one else has, and your body attacks it. Or you have something that everyone else has, but your body sees it as an intruder."

"Either way, I'm attacking myself."

His face softened, and the matter-of-factness faded away. Only compassion came through in his nod.

I'd learned a lot about interpersonal conflict in my job and school, but attacking myself—that was *inner*personal. I didn't have any classes in that.

The end of suffering was in sight. The doctor would fix me, and I'd rejoin the ranks of the normal. *What'll it be? A pill? A shot? Another IV bag to flow into the highway of fluid running through my hand?*

He stood from his wheeled stool, and my eyes followed the unfolding of his frame. He was even taller to me now, seer of my insides. Solver of the mystery plaguing and eluding me for the last seven years. He'd given my pain a name. "The bad news is..."

*No. No bad news.*

"We don't know what causes it, so there is *no cure*. We'll manage the symptoms as best we can with medication. You'll go into remission, you'll have flare-ups. It'll be a cycle of good days and bad days."

I nodded numbly. The words *no cure* pinballed off the inside of my skull. There was relief in being legit—a professional verification of my suspicion. My trip in and strip down, with a sleepless night on skritchy sheets, was not for naught.

The weight of his words pulled my head down into the pillow as we both resigned to this prognosis: Me with the problem, and him, after years of study and practice, still without a solution.

While he scribbled on his prescription pad, my mind scrambled to wrap around what he said. *It's still going to be with me. They can't take it away. They don't know how.*

Part of me wished I'd never come, that I'd stayed on Lori's couch with the cold washcloth and her warm words telling me everything would be alright. There I could pretend. There, I still had my denial, the distractions of an overstuffed life, and ambitions driving me to the top.

But most of all, I had the wistful intention that one day I would go to the doctor and they would make it all go away.

# GUT INSTINCTS

"This one's for prednisone," he said, handing me the first script. "You'll start on a high dose, get into remission. But it's a steroid, so we'll have to taper you off. Hopefully your body picks up the baton."

He handed me the other one. "Sulfasalazine. Eight pills, twice a day. You'll stay on these for the rest of your life. They make you burn easily, so stay out of the sun."

*For the rest of your life.* That phrase cut through anesthesia's haze. The sun—my joy, my therapy, my bronze badge of summer—was now my enemy.

*I* was my enemy.

It was a jagged little pill to swallow.

I looked back at the drawing on my bedside table. *Erase those dashes. Or at least smooth them. Tell me the worst is over, that I'll feel a whole lot better from here on out. Scribble something on that fancy notepad of yours, and make.it.stop.*

I sighed and looked back out the window, down to the street. A boy in a hoodie waited for the bus, listening to the Discman tucked into the side pocket of his backpack. A smartly dressed woman fought with the wind for her dry cleaning.

I longed to trade places with either one of them.

Had I done this to myself? Why was I attacking myself? The Dexatrim and dieting. . . sticking my finger down my throat. . . the valium overdose. . . the cutting—each memory flashed through me like an accusation.

No wonder my body hated me.

*This is my fault.*

His words stapled the scarlet letter of weirdness already pinned to my chest—Crohn's, *cha-chung*—disease, *cha-chung*. I had officially joined the fraternity of the pitiful.

"Soooo, here's the thing. . ." he mused.

Surprised, I oriented back towards his voice. *I thought he left.*

He'd paused at the door. "I seem to have two kinds of patients," he said, eyes far off. "One group believes everything I say and it's true for them, they suffer. The other group ignores me and they get better." He shrugged. "The only difference I can see between the two groups is a decision."

And just like that, he was gone.

*Is he serious?!* Like a cartoon character in free fall, I could suddenly run mid-air. I'd been given a life sentence. *But now it's more of a question?*

My nurse caught my dazed stare and smiled. "So," her tone invited, "have you decided which group you want to be in?"

"Uh. . . I think I like the sound of the second one." Half-laughing, half-asking permission. Gratitude rushed through me for my compassionate and competent guide, shepherding me through such rocky terrain. The doctor gave orders, but she helped me implement, teaching me tricks and tucking me in when I was raw and empty and scared.

She did not yell 'PSYCHE!' and then laugh maniacally, as if it were some cruel joke—like I was half-worried she might. Nor did she applaud me. "Good," she said, pulling a small notepad from her scrubs and scribbling something down. She tore the page and handed it to me. "Here's where you start."

And then she, too, exited the room.

As I watched her go, I wondered what she'd written. What little piece of wisdom would grant my reprieve? The location where this magical second group met and the secret password to give at the door?

I stared down at the words: *Fit for Life* by Harvey and Marilyn Diamond.

# GUT INSTINCTS

*A book?*
*A diet book?*

---

**Theme / Emotional Wound:** *Self-betrayal + internalized blame.* The moment your pain is given a name, it comes with a paradox: clarity and condemnation. The real shame wasn't Crohn's—but that I was attacking myself. That my body turned against me and I deserved it.

**Old Survival Pattern:** *Self-punishment through hyper-responsibility.* Even in diagnosis, your first instinct is to take the blame. To treat your problems like a moral failings. You can choose for it to be the moment where that survival pattern begins to unravel.

**Gut Instincts Healing Method Stage:** *Face → Feel.* You're no longer running. You're sitting face-to-face with the truth of your situation. This is the first step in your transformation. Inner wisdom rises to meet the moment and takes the wheel. Your power is not gone. If the grief that begins to surface is processed, agency is reborn.

**Reflection:**
In moments like these, our most significant act of courage is not to abandon ourselves. To remember that as messy and imperfect as we are, we are still worthy of love and we deserve support. Sometimes the power of decision happens by invitation and sometimes by rebellion. Either way, it's the first step towards change and no one can take it for us—but no one can stop us either. We alone make our choices and we must make them with intention. A crisis is a call to that action.

The nurse's book suggestion felt like a breadcrumb on the trail back to myself.

## Reader Reflections:

1. **Releasing Shame Around Illness.** Have I ever believed I caused my illness, pain, or struggle? What shame or blame am I ready to release?
2. **Untangling Identity from Productivity.** Do I associate my worth with my ability to be "good," "productive," or "in control"? How has this belief shaped my healing journey?
3. **Redefining the Meaning of Diagnosis.** What do I fear a diagnosis might say about me? What new meaning could I choose instead—one rooted in resilience, not shame?
4. **Stepping Into Healing with Courage.** What would it feel like to decide I'm capable of healing—even if I don't know how yet?

## Affirmation:

*I am the healer I've been waiting for.*

# GUT INSTINCTS

Scan the Code Below to View the Video for Chapter 18:
Or go to: https://youtu.be/kj29xrTbvJ0

# Chapter 19

# Another One Bites the Dust

### The Cycle of False Hope
When the solution becomes the trap, it's time to find another way.

> *You may encounter many defeats,*
> *but you must not be defeated.*
> ~Maya Angelou

A book seemed like a feeble offering for the big problem I had. Besides, it sounded like a dieting book, and everything I ate went right through me.

Armed with those sulfa-based pellets of hope and high-dose steroids, I checked out of my hospital room with a view and migrated back into my paused life, part of the world again.

The steroid prednisone worked wonders. I had energy and an appetite. Bathrooms stopped occupying the top spot in my awareness. I could focus more on the professor than the ticking time bomb of my bowels. My time didn't get hijacked by extended stays in a stall. I felt stronger and no longer surfed wave after wave of pain. I was more alert, worked more efficiently, and transitioned fluidly from class notes to case notes, with plenty of stamina to manage my ambitious schedule.

Steroids were a double-edged sword. They gave me back my appetite and energy, but it came with a steep cost—weight gain, mood swings, thinning skin, elevated blood pressure and blood sugar. Long-term use led to bone loss, adrenal shutdown, increased risk of fractures.

"You should wear a medical alert bracelet," the pharmacist advised. "It notifies emergency personnel in the event of a crisis that your body won't produce the adrenaline needed, and they'll need to compensate. That's why you wean off them slowly, so your body starts to do the job again."

The bracelet's thick silver links accessorized, and emphasized, the scarlet letter on my chest—moving me even farther from the normalcy I craved.

I'd lay it all out on the calendar, detailing how much to take and when: from 40mg a day to 30mg, then 20mg. Then break the twenty in half to ten, then ten every other day until it just quietly slipped out the back door in the middle of the night, closed it softly behind, and tiptoed away.

Then we waited, hoping my body would take over, grab the baton and run with it, and, along with those chained to the shade sulfa drugs, keep me in remission.

That's so not what happened.

I woke up into a nightmare of feverish bowels on fire and the familiar feeling of something clawing and gnawing its way out of me. Balled up into the fetal position, moans growing louder, waking up Josh.

I had failed.

"Want to go to the hospital?" his groggy words reached through the dark.

"No." I groaned as I counted, again, how long the spasms lasted.

"But should we go anyway?"

## GUT INSTINCTS

My silence was as close to a yes as he was going to get, and he took it. He kissed my forehead, his poking mustache adding punctuation to his love, and gently threw back the covers. In a gap between spasms, we fumbled through sleepiness for clothes, then drove the thirty minutes on curvy country roads in the pitch dark to the nearest emergency room.

There would be no standoff at the ER roundabout. I knew I was beat. I'd go in willingly. I was already semi-surrendered—the diagnosis burst my bubble of denial. I'd changed into the easy-access gown and crawled up onto the skritchy bed sheets enough times that it got a little easier each time.

But with a little less hope than the last time.

Instead of a scope, the young nurse perkily thrust a Styrofoam cup with a bendy straw at me. "Here's your milkshake." After one sip, it was clear—no one who actually drank it would ever call it that.

Then we waited. For the Barium sludge to fight its way through me and add contrast to my bowels for viewing on a TV-like monitor above my bed. The doctor flicked it on and my intestines lit up in grainy black and white, like a film noir. We were detectives searching for the smoking gun, again.

"See here," the ER doc pointed, drawing all eyes to my insides where a group of intestines was huddled off to the side. "They're moving away from the inflamed section over there," he pointed to what looked like a balloon animal after a toddler got hold of it.

"And over here," he pointed to the narrow sections, "you're about the width of a pencil."

If he saw the irony of a pencil being his pointer, he didn't let on.

It wasn't wasted on me. Comic relief was a commercial break from the drama, and I clung to any amount of respite

I could get. I feared that if I lost my sense of humor, I'd really be fucked. So I chuckled to myself, softly, so the distorted balloon animal didn't get offended.

The name of my disease now had a face. Seeing it demystified it and gave me a sense of participation in addition to the explanation. Throw in the dashes drawn through that picture by Doctor Cute & Confident, and I could better visualize my body's processing plant, better understand what we were dealing with.

The nurse hung a bag of steroids onto my pole and snapped in a line to join the IV fluids already flowing into my veins, pumping me full of the same steroids I'd just weaned off—and at a much higher dose.

"This should help you feel a whole lot better," she assured me.

It did, but only for a little while.

Again, I plotted it out on the calendar: 40, 30, 20, 10. I stepped back and stared longingly at the last two weeks, when there were no numbers—the great white space of hope.

*I'll get there again.*

I'd eventually get down to the low doses, crossing off the days and crossing my fingers as I made the jump from half a pill every other day to none.

Again, we'd end up in the emergency room in the middle of the night—why do these things always happen in the middle of the night? Each trip followed the same script: gown, needle prick, "milkshake," balloon animal.

Cue steroids. Hope. Repeat.

A routine as familiar as it was demoralizing.

There was nothing new to see and nothing new to do about it. They made me the same offer, with the same 'Hopefully it works this time' tagline. I accepted it with all the optimism I could muster, which was a little less than the last time.

While Josh drove those thirty miles back home, I looked out the window—a mix of desperation and devastation, and wondered to the trees blurring by. *Will it work this time? Will this be the last time we make this trip?*

Each time, the side effects came back stronger and faster. I couldn't eat enough to get full, at least not for long. I gained twice as much weight and twice as fast, and before I could even get back into my regular-sized clothes, I gained it again.

Steroids made me super alert during lectures, but by the time my fellow seniors and I spilled out into the hallway, my belly had burned through the before-class meal and was grumbling for more. It pleaded like the plant from *Little Shop of Horrors*, "Feeeed meeeeee." Foodprints gave me away, leaving a trail through my day—ketchup smudge on a textbook, bit of avocado on a shirt hem, dried soup crinkling up lecture notes.

Emotionally, I was a raw nerve. A white shirt washed with something red would send me spiraling. Someone chewing too loudly? Fury. Josh caught most of my flaring rage and he never fought back, which somehow made it worse.

Phone calls turned snarky, then combative. I'd slam the receiver down, seething. Later, I'd wonder: *Who am I?* I started calling it Bitchisone and feared I'd have no friends left. (Heck, *I* didn't even like myself a lot of the time.)

The shame was smothering.

This treatment of jack me up on steroids, wean me off, jack up, wean off, had all the characteristics of riding the carousel at the fair as a kid: horse moving up and down, platform going round and round, but you're going nowhere.

*There's the Tilt-O-Whirl... the balloon game... the corn dog stand...*

There's the IV prick... the 'milkshake'... doses scribbled on the calendar...

Hope draining. Size gaining.

And then there was that slip of paper on the fridge, wedged under a magnet from spring break somewhere.

---

**Theme / Emotional Wound:** *Disillusionment + Defeat.* Surface-level fixes can't offer sustainable relief because they don't get to the root cause. This chapter reveals the painful emotional cost of giving your authority to someone else and believing what didn't work before will work the next time. The real wound is in the looping: trying, failing, and fearing this might be all there is.

**Old Survival Pattern:** *Dependency on external authority/ solution-chasing.* There's a loop forming—do what they say, hope it works, crash when it doesn't. Meanwhile, your inner voice is being drowned out. You learn to follow orders instead of following instincts.

**Gut Instincts Healing Method Stage:** *Feel → Face.* This is where you fully *feel* the cost of this approach. You face the reality that the merry-go-round model isn't sustainable. You're not rejecting help—but you're starting to question what help actually looks like.

## Reflection:

It was also like riding a roller coaster—temporary healing highs, the stomach-dropping plunge of relapse, and the corkscrews eroding hope. The soul weariness of trying to heal within a system that's only offering survival.

Sometimes the scariest thing isn't the pain—it's the moment you realize the people meant to save you don't have a long-term plan. When you've done everything right but still end up in the ER at 3 a.m., you begin to wonder: *Is this all there is?* But even in the swirl of side effects, there's a flicker—your gut, your spirit—asking if there's another way.

## Reader Reflection:

1. **Recognizing the Loop of False Hope:** Where in my healing journey have I felt like I was going in circles? What patterns of chasing solutions have kept me feeling stuck rather than empowered?
2. **Questioning External Solutions:** What treatments or protocols gave me short-term relief but left me feeling depleted or dependent? What did those experiences teach me about my body's deeper needs?
3. **Healing Beyond Betrayal:** Have I ever felt betrayed by a system I trusted? How can I honor the tools I've tried without making them the whole story?

# Affirmation:

*I honor the past and I choose a new path.*
*I alone write my story.*

## JENNIFER JUNIPER

Scan the Code Below to View the Video for Chapter 19:
Or go to: https://youtu.be/_l-YkuTBJiw

## Chapter 20

# Bullet With Butterfly Wings

### Breaking the Cycle
True freedom begins when you stop repeating
the patterns that broke you.

*Freedom begins the moment you decide
not to let someone else define your story.
~Unknown*

The Smashing Pumpkins said it best—despite all my rage, I was still a rat in a cage. And in my Advanced Experimental Psychology class, I found myself watching literal rats in cages, frantically pressing a lever for a one-in-a-thousand chance at a food pellet.

*Like me, taking another round of prednisone with the hope of hitting the jackpot: remission.*

The Milgram Shock Experiment provided disturbing insights, prompting me to seek personal applications. Milgram had intended to explain the psychology of genocide during the Holocaust—his results hit much closer to home.

I couldn't stop thinking about it. How easily people obeyed authority, even at the expense of their own moral judgment. *Is that me? ... taking another dose of sulfasalazine— those orange pellets of promise looked like dangling carrots—*

*handed to me by someone in a white coat.* Midnight trips to the emergency room told me they weren't working, but I kept obeying anyway.

Dealing with my own fuckedupness had been the one certainty I'd counted on when deciding to pursue a psychology degree, but I hadn't anticipated learning the huge role my subconscious played in determining my thoughts and beliefs while preparing for a career.

A career I'd been fortunate enough to jump-start as a very part-time, grant-funded Parent Aide position with the Department of Social Services. The eagerness to burst into my field and start changing the world turned into elation when I spotted the listing in the classifieds: *Degree preferred, but not required.* As a senior I was close to the finish line, but in the professional world I still had a few laps to go.

The job was just ten hours a week, helping at-risk parents build skills and connect them with resources to prevent foster care placement for their kids. Ten hours I didn't have to waitress. Ten hours that gave me a real job title and a foot in the door.

The office was softly lit—no harsh fluorescents, just lamps warmly glowing at two desks with a third wedged in. Empty. Waiting.

"Are you a parent?" My potential supervisor's eyes said it before her words did—she didn't think I was the right person for the job.

I glanced at the desk, and already pictured myself there. "I think that's illegal to ask (I knew it was, but hoped the Bitchisone didn't make me come off too strong) but I'll answer anyway. I'm not a parent, but I have *been parented*, and I can tell from a child's point of view what constitutes good and bad parenting. I'll come from the perspective of an affected child."

## GUT INSTINCTS

I continued sizing up the office as she sized me up. I'd have to buy a lamp. *Would I get a business card?*

A week later, the desk was mine. I slid my hand over the desk's smooth surface, opening the drawers just to hear them glide. Clicked on my new lamp like flipping a switch inside myself. This was mine. A real job. A place in the world, a caseload. No apron. No tray. Just file folders and a purpose.

I visited living rooms where cycles of trauma held families in its orbit. The parents weren't monsters. They were exhausted and ill-equipped—trying to parent without ever being properly parented themselves.

I taught them simple tools: how to encourage instead of criticize, use consequences instead of punishment, how to listen instead of lash out.

As I taught them, something shifted in me. The compassion I was modeling seeped inward. I began to hear my inner voice—the child I once was—more clearly. And for the first time, I didn't shut her down.

It was one thing to study trauma in textbooks, but quite another to witness its staying power across generations. Each parent had different intentions, but they reverted to their programmed factory settings when stressed.

I saw it so clearly. My mother's apology after one of her abusive eruptions—'I'll do better, I promise'—mirrored the cycles I saw in the parents I worked with. They meant well. They wanted to change. But they couldn't.

I empathized more than I cared to admit.

The parallels of my upbringing and personal battle to break the cycle accumulated right along with the miles to and from those home visits. Educating them about the effects of abuse on their children, empowering them with healthier ways to communicate—altered the inner workings of my machine as well.

Helping others helped me. Got me out of my head, absorbed with my problems and the lack of solutions. Offering optimism and encouragement around new thoughts and behaviors—and celebrating the results—smoothed and softened the strictness that'd left its imprint on my psyche and soul.

Being a Parent Aide turned out to be a lot like crafting with glitter. Glitter doesn't just stay where you put it; glitter gets everywhere. It's in the carpet, in your hair, you catch glints out of the corner of your eye from the residency it's taken up on your lashes.

Throughout my entire childhood, I fought to be heard. Now, teaching parents to listen to their kids, something shifted. My inner voice grew louder, clearer, more insistent. I began to hear myself in a way I never had before.

---

**Theme / Emotional Wound:** *Powerlessness + obedience to authority.* You realize you've been following orders that don't serve you on autopilot, trapped inside someone else's "shoulds." There's grief and anger here—not just at them, but at yourself. And underneath all that: a secret longing to take your life back.

**Old Survival Pattern:** *External validation + blind trust in authority.* Deferring to people in positions of power. The survival pattern here is 'outsourcing to survive' and trusting others over your own body, your own knowing, and your own voice.

**Gut Instincts Healing Method Stage:** *Face + Follow.* You're facing systems that failed you. And you're following something new: your purpose, your self-trust, your sacred NO. This chapter is a slow-burning ignition.

**Reflection:**
Sometimes the hardest cages to leave are the ones we don't even know we're in. Systems. Beliefs. Protocols. "Roles." We shrink to fit them. We obey because it's what good people do. But transformation requires rebellion—against the idea that someone else knows better. When you begin to listen inward, you become your own authority. That's where freedom lives.

## Reader Reflections:

1. **Reclaiming Inner Leadership.** Where in my life am I waiting for someone else to fix me, lead me, or give me permission? What would it feel like to take one small step without waiting for outside validation?
2. **Listening to the Inner Voice.** Do I silence my inner voice out of fear of being wrong, rude, or irresponsible? When have I known the truth inside me but doubted it because of outside pressure?
3. **Redefining Authority.** Have I mistaken compliance for healing? What's one "authority" (person, book, belief system) I've followed that may no longer serve me—and what new source of guidance am I ready to trust instead?

## Affirmation:

*I have all the permission I need to trust myself.*

# JENNIFER JUNIPER

Scan the Code Below to View the Video for Chapter 20:
Or go to: https://youtu.be/v84KXvj-Hq4

## Chapter 21

# Start Me Up

**It's Not *What* You are Eating, But *When***
Those first baby steps create massive leaps down the road.

*Small shifts in your thinking and small changes in your energy can lead to massive alterations in your end result.*
~Kevin Michel

*F*it *for Life—sounds like a diet book*, my mind harrumphed every time I opened the fridge, which meant it harrumphed a lot. *Could a book like that really be the answer the nurse gave to my problem?* My intestines turned food into scissors. Paper can't beat scissors—every second grader knows that.

I was already drowning in books—textbooks, notebooks, planners—and fighting the clock for time. I needed fast relief and an easier way.

A swallow-a-few-pills-and-get-on-with-your-day way.

But that wasn't easy, and it wasn't working, and I wasn't getting on. I was still doing battle with a body that battled itself. My uncertainty warred with my curiosity until I finally made a what-have-you-got-to-lose move. I snatched the paper off the fridge, grabbed the car keys, and headed to the bookstore.

# JENNIFER JUNIPER

With its cornucopia of raw fruits on the front cover and permanent weight-loss promise on the back, *Fit for Life* looked to be exactly the diet book I suspected it was.

I opened it anyway, daring it to prove me wrong.

Skimming past the usual suspects—*Principles, Theories, Protein, and Exercise* until Chapter 12 stopped me cold: *You Are What You Think You Are.*

According to Harvey and Marilyn Diamond (and science), we could consciously direct our cells to do what we wanted them to do. We were, in fact, already sending constant messages and commands to our cells which they carried out diligently.

Then came the boldest line yet: *The body will bring about whatever result the conscious mind desires.*

Whoa.

I'd been learning about the mind driving behavior, but *could it . . . also . . . direct my health?* Just entertaining the possibility pushed my brain to the border. In trepidation, it peered over into the foreign land where this powerful concept staked its flag.

A past scene played from memory. Me in the hospital bed, Doctor Cute and Confident in the doorway, 'The only difference I can see between the two groups is a decision.' Hadn't I declared my choice to be in the group that got better to the nurse? *Was this the admission ticket, stuck on my fridge the whole time?*

My skepticism gave way to optimism inside the frame of such radical ideas. But radical was what I needed—some thinking outside the box I was trapped in. I flipped back to the Foreword, where one sentence awaited to seal the deal. *Even the slightest change, the least little consistent effort, and healthy fitness ensues.*

*I can do that. I can make a slight change.* I kept reading.

# GUT INSTINCTS

Different foods digested differently. Fruit moved quickest, taking just thirty minutes. Nuts took hours. Meat even longer. Proper combining was key. Only foods with similar processing times should be eaten together. Otherwise, the faster foods sit atop the slow ones, rotting and gassing up the joint (those gas bubbles have to come out somewhere).

Apparently, my beloved sandwich was a digestive disaster.

Already juggling so much, I didn't know where I'd find the time to read about—much less implement—a new way of eating. I was a grab-and-goer—eating while driving, studying, or chewing a flattened granola bar between classes that I found at the bottom of my bookbag.

But that sentence from the Foreword kept circling. *Even the slightest change...*

I looked for an easy entry point. *Fruit, with its high-water content and fast digestion, should be eaten alone and in the morning, when the body is in detox mode.*

There it was.

Eating only fruit for breakfast actually gave me time. No cooking. No toasting. I grabbed bananas and blueberries for the drive to campus, stuffed grapes into the side pocket of my book bag to pop in my mouth during class. My tummy stopped gurgling. My energy lifted. My brain tracked lectures more easily.

Small shift, big ripple.

Hope returned from its hiatus and I renewed my commitment to the second group.

At first, food combining felt like another pile of rules on top of an already complicated life. But when I saw the results, I realized it wasn't about restriction at all. It was about support and giving my body the conditions it needed to heal.

The bread on my lunch sandwich got replaced by lettuce. Sometimes I ditched the meat altogether. My stomach pain dulled. I wasn't so gassy. My internal processing plant finally caught a break. Encouragement turned to empowerment. It felt like I was in charge again.

A fire was lit, and the pages of that book fanned the flame.

I read it faster. Made more changes. Red meat took up to a week to digest, so the following Saturday night, when Josh and I went to our usual Surf-n-Turf at the supper club on the lake, I surveyed my prime rib differently.

*I don't think my system can afford that kind of time.*

"Would you want to trade me? My prime rib for your lobster tail?" I asked coyly.

"You know the difference between parsley and pussy?" he said, already grinning, teasing me with the green garnish.

I rolled my eyes. *Here it comes.*

"*Nobody* eats parsley." His shoulders bouncing with laugh-ter, he moved the sprig to the coaster under his Brandy Old Fashioned.

I tried not to laugh. Tried.

Always in support of anything that made me feel better, he slid his plate toward mine. "So you want a Surf-n-Surf instead, do ya?" laughing and stabbing my steak while I scooped up his crustacean.

"Thanks, babe. You're the best." I puckered my lips in an air kiss.

"Can I get that in writing for the next time I put the toilet paper on wrong?" he winked.

Coming from a world where people were always leav-ing—or showing up out of nowhere—Josh's steady presence gave me my first solid foundation. I'd never felt so safe. He never judged, never fought back. He just wanted me happy.

# GUT INSTINCTS

Whatever it took to get me well, he'd do that. All I had to do was ask.

Switching to the turkey versions of bacon and burgers was easy. I swore my intestines sighed at the reprieve. I reached for veggies and dip at the school café. Carried trail mix in my purse and kept a backup stash in my glove box.

With each shift, my bowels worked better. I didn't race to the bathroom—I strolled. No more pulling over to poop in the bushes on the way home from school.

I'd been given a taste of feeling better, and wanted the whole enchilada.

*God, I miss enchiladas.*

---

**Theme / Emotional Wound:** *Drowning in solutions that don't solve.* When results become unreliable and expertise keeps failing, hope turns exhausting—every new approach feels like another weight instead of a life raft. We're shifting from stuck to stirred.

**Old Survival Pattern:** *Only dramatic shifts count.* When you've needed big solutions just to survive, gradual improvement feels insufficient—almost insulting. But healing means learning to replace the inner voice that scoffs at "baby steps" with one that celebrates each small victory as evidence of real change.

**Gut Instincts Healing Method Stage:** *Follow. Aligned action.* Taking small steps that feel right even without understanding, choosing support over restriction, and letting results build while trusting in your own guidance.

## Reflection:

I didn't realize it at the time, but something ancient in me was starting to wake up.

A spark I thought had gone out. Aliveness that wasn't tied to productivity, safety, or being "good." Just the raw, humming knowing that there was more for me than symptom management and self-denial.

Back then, I wasn't just hungry for food—I was starving for feeling. For energy, sensuality, for permission to want. Maybe you know that ache, too. Perhaps you've been surviving so long that you forgot what it feels like to *desire* something beyond relief.

But desire is sacred. Pleasure is data. And aliveness is your birthright, not a luxury. What if your healing isn't about going back to how you used to be, but forward into more of who you really are?

Sometimes, the most minor changes are the most sacred. Stay Curious. Stay Open.

## Reader Reflection:

1. **Releasing Perfectionism Around Healing.** Where have I waited for the "perfect" moment to make a change? What slight shift could I try today—without needing to commit to everything?
2. **Listening to the Body's Natural Rhythms.** How does my body respond to different kinds of food or rhythms? What patterns or signals am I ignoring because they don't fit a certain "ideal"?
3. **Questioning Inherited Beliefs.** What beliefs have I inherited about what healing "should" look like? Where did those beliefs come from—and are they still serving me?

GUT INSTINCTS

## Affirmation:

*I honor the wisdom of my body
and trust that even the smallest positive choices
bring me closer to well-being and harmony.*

Scan the Code Below to View the Video for Chapter 21:
Or go to: https://youtu.be/adGdLpQ706U

# Chapter 22

# I Want to Break Free

### The Power of Belief
Liberation from old identities.

*Some things have to be believed to be seen.*
~Anonymous

I drove to my next doctor's appointment emboldened by belief. In *me* and my body's ability to come back online, digestive-wise. Buzzing with hope I sat on the edge of my waiting room chair, ready to share the progress I'd made.

My new gastroenterologist was closer to home than the one who diagnosed me, but—I would soon learn—worlds away from the two-group paradigm I was operating under.

His nurse looked up from my open chart, forehead crinkled, pen suspended. "How do you spell Crohn's again?"

I offered it dutifully, like a good little patient. Seismically, I shifted. I was acutely aware of my freakness when out and about in the world, but being a weirdo within a system designed to treat anomalies turned the alienation up a notch.

Quickly, I recapped for the doctor—Doctor #5—my failed attempts to wean off the steroids and the middle-of-the-night trips to the emergency room. I briefly explained the food combining theory, how it worked, and how it helped.

How eating only fruit in the morning boosted my energy levels, making me more alert and giving my belly an easy start to the day. "I think it's making me better."

He didn't smile or ask questions. The skepticism in his eyes locked on me in silent judgment of my efforts. "You should be peeling those apples," his flat tone dismissing everything I'd shared.

My heart sank. "I don't have time to peel apples." Couldn't he see how much this was helping me?

"Fruits and vegetables have a lot of fiber. You could form a blockage," he said, tapping his index finger on my file folder—thick with test and scope results, the late-night airings of *My Inflamed Intestines*, every prescription of the protocol, and all the times it didn't work. "You should be eating what's called a low-residue diet: white bread, white rice, fruits and veggies should be cooked well. Baby food when you're in a flare."

"Blech! I don't like any of that stuff. But I'm eating healthy..."

"You're eating healthy for a normal person," said Doctor Skeptical. "But not for someone with severe Crohn's."

*Normal.* The mere mention of that driving force of a word, my holy grail, made my brain's neon sign flicker and hum to life. *Oh, but I want to be normal...*

Pushing aside the residual battle cry of my childhood, I focused on my new, more prominent need to break out of this cycle of managing symptoms and failing repeatedly. It didn't make any sense to stop what was working, especially when the other treatment *wasn't*. Maybe I couldn't explain why eating the *Fit for Life* way helped alleviate my symptoms, but I could sure feel it.

And I trusted it.

"I'm afraid it's the only treatment we've got." Dr. Skeptical said as he handed me another prescription and headed for the door, leaving me with the sting of his indifference, his pin

# GUT INSTINCTS

prick of doubt stuck in my balloon of hope *It's not the only treatment I've got.*

Doing the same thing over and over again, expecting different results, was the definition of insanity. The doctor's loyalty to an ineffective approach and his dismissal of the working one fueled my determination to keep exploring alternatives. The whole visit watered the seed of defiance taking root in me. If they wouldn't celebrate my progress, *I* would. And I'd keep searching for those who could.

Walking out of his office, something shifted. His indifference lit a fire. If I wanted to heal, I couldn't keep relying on people who couldn't even see me. I needed to trust myself more.

I summoned the memory of Doctor Cute & Confident and my hospital nurse. I received guidance from the piece of paper torn from her notebook, fueled by the promise of the second group—as well as all the treatment failures—I had a hunch I was onto something. My hunches had helped me before...

I'd listened to my gut, not showing up to business school. The quiet space of a semester with no one to answer to but myself, nudged me onto a new career path. I chose a psychology major on a hunch. There were two universities to consider when moving to Neshkoro with Josh, both equally far away. I chose the University of Wisconsin–Stevens Point for the very sound and logical reason of the school's colors—purple and gold. Purple was my favorite. Purple meant Prince, and Prince, well, Prince was perfection. (Stevens Point was also home to Point Brewery, and at twenty-two, I'd already developed an affinity for above-average beer.)

Those hunches were paying off.

A campus chosen on color and beer revealed a bigger significance and broader applications. Almost as if something in me had known something. I walked past a wall declaring an emphasis on health and wellness, learned of pioneering degrees focusing on holistic approaches that integrated physical, mental, and social well-being.

I felt less lonely knowing my school had my back.

A small food co-op sat kitty-corner to campus, calling me to explore and further experiment with the powerful healing properties found in nature and food.

As I pushed open the door, the smell of fresh herbs and baked goods wafted around me in warm embrace, whispering, 'You belong here.' A bakery case filled with good-for-you muffins and samosas made from ingredients kissed by Mother Nature beckoned me further inside.

For the first time, I felt my strategy not only validated but celebrated. With each visit, I added a new thing to the once-new, now old stuff I was doing. I switched to water processed decaf and traded drive-thrus for organic, plant based grab-n-go's.

I could make all these changes because I felt supported. The proximity of the co-op to campus, the ease of its offerings, the knowledgeable and sympathetic staff, who started as guides and became confidants.

The more they knew about my condition, the more informed and dialed-in their ideas became. No prescriptions. No side effects. No judgment. And most importantly, they believed like I did that total healing was possible.

"Sprouting tricks a seed into thinking it's growing. That shift activates enzymes and unlocks nutrients," one staff shared.

"Fermentation partially breaks the food down *before* you even eat it. That means less work for your gut." Another one offered on another day. Sugar was inflammatory and addictive, so I bought a bag of honey-sweetened granola to munch on when striding between classes.

Classes that were more fascinating now that I wasn't only preparing for my future and my field, but also extracting any current benefits applicable to what I was going through personally. The Placebo Effect would've been a fascinating concept on its own, but its application to my plight was what really excited me.

"Two groups were given the same-looking pill, and both were told it was medicine." The researcher in the lab coat on the video reported dryly. "One group got real medicine, the other a sugar pill—the placebo. Seventy percent of those in the placebo group got better."

My mind swirled around his findings, making me almost choke on a grape. *Seventy percent! How's that even possible?*

The man in the white coat and clunky black framed glasses answered back. "The power of belief is statistically significant in the treatment of disease."

I had that! I had the power of belief. I believed in miracles—the Bible was full of them: burning bushes, a blind man seeing, the parting of the Red Sea. Dad waking up from a coma when they didn't think he'd make it through the night was miraculous—gaining back six inches of once-paralyzed muscle, a miracle on top of a miracle. God made a scene in the grass when I was a bawling little girl, distraught and desperate for my dad to come get me.

If belief alone could heal 70% of the placebo group, what might happen if I combined belief with actions that felt aligned with my body's needs? A spark reignited my hope. My belief wasn't just a soft, intangible idea—it held power. It was *statistically significant.*

*I believed I was qualified to be a Parent Aide, visualized myself sitting at that empty desk, and now it's mine.*

Memories of a clumsy childhood flicked me back further to cuts and bruises, and my mother's consistent remedy: 'Want me to kiss it and make it better?' The kiss *would* make it better. Older me used it on the kids I babysat for, and it worked for them, too. 'Kiss it and make it better' didn't have the slightest bit of medical validity, but it worked.

Despite following every prevention tip, the cycle of UTIs and yeast infections continued. My body was a battleground I couldn't escape—or claim victory on. Josh and mine's trips to the ER diversified into peeing liquid fire into a cup and waiting in agony for a nurse to confirm what I already knew.

"You've got a urinary tract infection," the doctor announced with pride.

"Yes, I know."

He handed me a prescription for antibiotics and turned to leave, case closed, but I pressed him, wanting to know the cause and how I could prevent them.

"They're often brought on by intercourse. Your partner's fluids are foreign, and the urethra is so close to the vaginal opening." He looked at Josh, then back at me. "Your body will eventually get used to him, and they'll stop."

Josh and I locked eyes in disbelief. "But we've been together for three years."

The doctor shrugged. "The best prevention is urinating after sex."

I already jumped up mid-afterglow, so I started doing it sooner, only to end up in the ER peeing fire into another cup.

I'd jump up even sooner—another UTI.

Sooner.

Another.

As if that wasn't enough excitement, I started getting yeast infections, turning the intake process into a 'Which hole are you here for' kind of situation. My ER takeout order cycled between steroids, antibiotics, and plungers of white cream.

Then, to really mix it up, I developed an insanely painful Bartholin's cyst and could barely walk. The night after it was lanced and drained, I soaked in a warm bath wondering why my body was revolting. *Again.* The more I tried to push my life forward, the more health issues arose to pull me backward.

Trying to get better made me sicker and sicker.

I sank further into the tub.

Seeing *Jaws* as a kid, it didn't stay on the TV screen. It followed me into lakes, pools, even baths became scary. The water was never neutral again. I'd outgrown the terror trigger, but the rebel yell seemed pretty apropos...

'We're gonna need a bigger boat.'

---

**Theme / Emotional Wound:** *Fighting to be heard.* When what's working for you gets dismissed by others, you're caught between trusting your own experience and needing external validation—forced to choose between being "compliant" or moving forward.

**Old Survival Pattern:** *Authority over intention.* When others disagree with your lived experience, they must be right and you must be wrong. But growth means discovering the expertise without the curiosity isn't wisdom and your instincts have guided you well before.

**Gut Instincts Healing Method Stage:** *Filter → Follow.* Intuitive discernment → aligned, self-honoring action. Sifting through misinformation, tuning out outside noise. Trusting your instincts, building a custom path, and refusing to abandon what *feels* right.

**Reflection:**
I walked into that appointment hoping to be seen. Instead, I got a cookie-cutter protocol and a box I no longer fit in. I didn't know it then, but that moment of dismissal cracked something open in me.

It didn't crush my hope—it rerouted it. That was the beginning of trusting my gut in ways that would change everything.

Maybe you've been there, too. Shut down. Talked over. Given answers that didn't fit the questions you were asking. But what if their disbelief doesn't mean your truth is wrong? What if their story has nothing to do with yours?

You're allowed to keep going, even when they stop listening. You're allowed to celebrate your progress, even if no one else does. You're allowed to trust what works—even if it doesn't make sense on paper.

Sometimes freedom starts as a quiet knowing: *This path isn't mine anymore.*

Seeing *Jaws* too young was unfiltered input that I had to metabolize on my own tiny terms. I had to grow armor when what I really needed was attunement. Textbook nervous system imprinting disguised as edginess. And when no one's modeling what safety feels like, mistrust becomes the baseline. Not because you're cynical—but because you're *sensitized.*

Gen X was collectively thrown to the wolves, but I was particularly sensitive. My wiring wasn't built for numbness— it was built for *noticing*. And when you grow up noticing *everything* but being told nothing matters, it fractures you a bit. It resurfaces later as dysregulation. That means you're safe enough *now* for the nervous system to finally say, "Okay. Can we deal with this?"

**Reader Reflection:**

1. **Reclaiming Inner Authority.** This chapter marks a turning point: no longer deferring to external experts but asserting our right to choose what feels aligned. It's about trusting yourself—even when others don't. Where have you handed your power over to experts—even when your gut said otherwise? When was the last time you silenced your truth to seem agreeable or "compliant"? Can you recall a moment when your body screamed 'yes' while someone in authority said 'no'?
2. **Belief as a Healing Tool.** Belief isn't naïve—it's *active*. Hope becomes a form of resistance. Agency becomes a path toward wellness. What do you believe about your ability to heal?

    Is it limiting—or liberating? When have you witnessed the power of belief—yours or someone else's—create real change? What would shift if you allowed belief to take up more space than doubt?
3. **The Friction of Awakening.** As we step into our truth, we collide with systems built on hierarchy. This is the messy middle—between clarity and compliance, between truth and the risk of rejection. Have you ever known something deeply but felt afraid to say it out loud? What does it feel like when you start trusting yourself more than someone with authority? Where are you currently experiencing the discomfort of growth?

JENNIFER JUNIPER

## Affirmation:

*I give myself permission to trust myself.
My body knows. I know.
That's enough.*

Scan the Code Below to View the Video for Chapter 22:
Or go to: https://youtu.be/K5vJKFNyMA0

## Chapter 23

# Let's Get (Meta)Physical

**Getting to the Root**
Real healing happens when you stop treating the surface and start discovering the source.

*You become what you think about.*
*~Earl Nightingale*

I clutched my book bag like a shield, heart pounding, brain disbelieving what I was about to ask. "Do you have any books on the mind-body connection?" I whispered to the librarian, like I was asking for porn.

Self-help was emerging, but far from mainstream. I readied my lie on my lips—'I'm doing research for a class'—in case she looked at me funny. The Placebo Effect haunted the halls of my mind. I heard its echo when I was trying to sleep and the steroids wouldn't let me.

The librarian thought for a moment and pointed. "There are a few books about that over there."

Under graying fluorescent lights, on a dusty, gray metal shelf, a slice of rainbow shone. Tipping my head to the side, I drank in the spine of *You Can Heal Your Life* by Louise Hay.

My mind choked on that big gulp of an idea. *Wait a minute. Does my whole life need healing?* I took a deep breath and pulled out the rest of the rainbow heart, a little afraid of what I might find. Then I flipped it over.

*If we are willing to do the mental work, almost anything can be healed.* That line stopped me cold.

Healed. Not just 'managed' or lived with. Not good days and bad days, seesawing between remission and flare-ups. Not taking medication for the rest of my life, clinging to the hope that I'll be able to do the things I want, and half holding my breath waiting for science to make a breakthrough.

The steroids and sulfasalazine were looking like a pair of dice rolling around in my palm. With every swallow, I gambled on a small slice of normalcy. Most days, I lost.

Snowmobiling (*shake*). It's an Olympic sport, getting out of a snowsuit mid-flare, your intestines set to 'firehouse.' Not fun. Commuting to campus (fingers crossed). Running to the bathroom (praying I made it.) I bargained with my bowels and braced myself for the worst through lectures, study sessions, tests, home visits, intakes, meetings, boating, weddings, restaurants.

On Sunday drives with sunbeams streaming through the T-tops of Josh's Thunderbird.

Safely tucked between two walls of books, I let out some leash on my beliefs and entertained this new possibility. Tepidly, I opened the front cover. The Dedication pulled me in further: *May this offering help you find the place within where you know your own self-worth—the part of you that is pure love and self-acceptance.*

I wasn't too sure there was a place in me like that, but Hay's warm words of possibility were a refreshing change from the cold, clinical skepticism of my doctor visits and lured me in further. The Foreword mentioned a reference guide to probable mental patterns behind a presenting disease.

## GUT INSTINCTS

Flipping further, I found Louise's story of being sexually abused as a child and the correlation of getting diagnosed with cancer in the vaginal area later in life.

A manifestation that made perfect sense, she thought.

I looked up at the poked hole patterning of the ceiling tiles above me and that theory and wondered how mine could be that simple. Intestinal abuse wasn't even a thing. *I suppose I abused them—making myself vomit, starving myself, taking diet pills.*

Turning to the reference guide, I found no Crohn's listed in the *Problem* column. *Of course.* My eyes flitted about, landing a few alphabetically aligned spaces above: *Colitis. Close enough.* Following along with my finger to the middle column, *Probable Cause,* I read, 'Over-exacting parents. Feelings of oppression and defeat. Great need for affection.'

Words that hit me right between the eyes. I trembled a little from the impact.

All I could do was stare forward, stunned, while a whole slew of memories uncorked themselves: hearing my mother often brag about having me potty trained by eighteen months; how she convinced the school principal to let me start kindergarten a year early; the clicking of her tongue in dismay at an A- on my report card.

I felt a heady mix of anger, grief, and validation. The dashes drawn by Doctor Cute & Confident looked different to me in light of Hay's suggested causation. *Did my intestines crack under the pressure?*

*Great need for affection.* I thought back to all the times I chased parents who didn't want to be there for me. The nights I cried myself to sleep, missing my daddy. All those times I wanted and waited for him to be in my life, to act like a dad. All the things I never said but I should've, because I was afraid he'd go away again.

He left anyway.

In the middle of my mind's free fall, I latched onto the third column's *New Thought Pattern*. *I love and approve of myself. I create my own joy. I choose to be a winner in life.* My mind opened like a parachute.

Would healing stem from transformed beliefs about myself?

A brief paragraph under the word *Treatment* held a bold premise. The boldest. *I am one with the very Power that created me, and this Power has given me the power to create my own circumstances.*

My brain bucked at such words, offering counter-arguments of all the circumstances I was pretty sure I *hadn't* created. Exhibit A: Growing up without a dad. Exhibit B: Being sent to private school. Exhibit C: My stomach problems. *No, I'm sure I didn't create any such circumstances.* I had, in fact, pleaded and prayed for them to change.

But I also knew I had created some of my circumstances: getting out of my hometown, landing the Parent Aide job, even scoring spots in full classes (I showed up anyway, in case someone dropped out).

And I knew I didn't want to be a passive participant in my healing. I craved empowered certainty.

I turned another page.

*When we really love ourselves, everything in our lives works.* (The mention of self-love made me cringe.) *We create every so-called 'illness' in our body.*

So-called? 'Illness'?? I bristled. I considered stuffing the book back into the gap on the shelf. But something stopped me. Radical seemed to be the new normal. I welcomed the reprieve from the mundane repetition of an ineffective treatment plan.

# GUT INSTINCTS

Not everything landed. But what did made me feel seen, not studied.

*No person, no place, and no thing has any power over us, for we are the only thinkers in our minds.*

I liked the sound of that. I sensed the freedom it offered. Inside the front cover, I found a copyright date of 1984. The same year my symptoms started. *Maybe it is a sign?* Desperate for a true solution to my situation, I took it as one.

When a culprit is still at large, a good detective investigates any possible leads. *What have I got to lose?*

*You Can Heal Your Life*'s lavender-hued neighbor called me back to the shelf. I ran my finger along *Love, Medicine, & Miracles*, letting the synergy of those three words sink in. The subtitle continued: *Lessons Learned About Self-Healing from a Surgeon's Experience with Exceptional Patients.*

The back cover got right to the point. *The truth is: love heals. Miracles happen to exceptional patients every day—patients who have the courage to love, those who have the courage to work with their doctors to participate in and influence their own recovery.*

Savoring Dr. Siegel's words risked me being late to class. Not savoring them was risky, too—prolonged suffering, more trips to the ER, my future plans jeopardized further.

I compromised, quickly skimming the introduction. Siegel told the story of Norman Cousins diagnosed with tuberculosis as a teen and spending six months at a sanitarium. Cousins reported the patients dividing themselves into two groups: those who were confident they would beat back the disease and be able to resume normal lives, and those who resigned themselves to a prolonged and even fatal illness.

The boys in the first group had a much higher percentage of being discharged as cured than the kids in the second group, Cousins concluded.

*My second group compatriots!* I had company, even if only on paper. The story wrapped around me in a cloak of solidarity.

Siegel spoke of cancer patients *not dying like they were supposed to,* an idea that both made me smile and made me more curious. Envious. I wanted to beat the odds! The patients hadn't gone home intending not to die, but rather with the attitude: If I only have one year to live, how do I want to live it?

Not dying was simply a side effect of living a life one loved, fearlessly and without apology.

Wheels turned and gears clicked in my mind. We'd been going at my belly through my belly, but these cancer patients were affecting their disease with their hearts.

*Go from WHY ME? to TRY ME!* The book continued.

The price of admission to the second group had been a decision.

I held the book to my chest, against a heart buoyed by fresh possibility, camaraderie, and a crack at total freedom instead of living on a rug that could be pulled out from under me at any time. My heart ached for a doctor like Bernie Siegel.

My doctor was more stringent and didn't want to hear about anything innovative, waving off the results I was getting. He clearly was not of the 'patients participating in and influencing their own recovery' persuasion.

Just the opposite.

There I was, between classes, between two metal rows of books, and between two schools of thought: traditional modern medicine's dire prognosis and these new age, metaphysical, mind-body connection concepts. I wondered again if a book could be the solution to my problem.

But mostly, I wondered what it would mean if my condition wasn't permanent.

# GUT INSTINCTS

*Just as disease can be used to heal a life, so can this book.*
I raced off to class, accompanied by Louise Hay and Dr. Siegel and activated by the stories of those who'd walked before me. The idea of decision stayed with me, not just as a concept but as a challenge. Could I decide to heal even if I didn't fully believe it was possible?

I couldn't wait to read more.

* * *

Closing in on graduation, I realized my final semester classes were preparing me for more than just a career. They introduced me to something I'd overlooked in my drive to help others—the vital role of self-care to avoid burnout. My professor, as fond of analogies as I was, demonstrated it this way: "What the stewardess tells you about putting the oxygen mask on yourself before helping others, that applies to this job as well."

He dimmed the lights and popped in a video tracking a woman across various therapists employing different modalities. I welcomed any animation of the curriculum, but the video did more than bring our textbook to life—it exposed my own psyche.

The patient and I shared some traits. She grappled with the weight of the past pressing on her present. She too, had tried to change her behavior on her own with lackluster results. Her comment at the end reminded me of the power of supported self-examination to liberate us from the patterns of the past. "It felt nice to be truly listened to. I feel like I know myself more and better understand why I do some of the things I do and how to change."

*I want that. I want to be listened to and understand what's driving my behavior, so I can change.*

I'd been focusing a lot on what I was eating, but what about what was eating me? The professor's permission for self-care, coupled with the metaphysical causation of over-exacting parents, made me wonder. *What if, under the auspices of being ambitious, I'd really just internalized the high expectations from my childhood because I couldn't find the off-switch?*

After class, I went back to the Student Health Services building—this time to make an appointment with a therapist. Maybe the bravest thing wasn't fixing me. It was letting someone see me—mess and all.

---

**Core Theme / Emotional Wound:** *Powerlessness + inherited perfectionism.* This chapter is about realizing healing requires more than effort, obedience, or intellect. Underneath the physical struggle is a deeper emotional inheritance: being over-pressured to perform, to be "exceptional," to get it right. And beneath that, the heartbreak of a little kid who still craves affection and approval. The wound is in the belief that *worth is tied to perfection and performance.*

**Old Survival Pattern:** *Intellectualization + Overachievement as survival.* Trying to solve your problem the way you've been trained to solve everything: through studying, compliance, data, external validation. But here, we hit a spiritual wall: healing isn't only about logic. It's about *liberating the inner terrain*—our thoughts, patterns, pain, and the permission we give ourselves.

We're slowly waking up to the truth that what's eating us isn't just physical—it's emotional, spiritual, and ancestral.

# GUT INSTINCTS

**Gut Instincts Healing Method Stage:** *Filter → Follow → Filter.* We're beginning to sort through conflicting paradigms: mainstream intellect vs. metaphysical wisdom. Learning to discern what resonates, even when it's radical or uncomfortable.

*Follow:* Taking a concrete step like booking a therapy appointment, not because someone tells us to, but because something in us *knows* it's time. It's intuitive action rooted in self-inquiry. Discernment becomes decision. Seeking answers transforms into starting to trust our own.

## Reflection:
I didn't know exactly what I was searching for when I walked into that library. But I knew I needed more than another traditional take. I needed something that spoke to my gut, not just my symptoms. Something that reminded me that healing was still within my grasp.

At the time, I didn't know if I believed what I was reading. But I knew I was tired of believing I was broken. Sometimes healing doesn't begin with certainty. It begins with a question. Maybe you're holding an idea you're not sure about yet—but part of you whispers, *What if it's true?*

What if your thoughts have power? What if your body responds to belief just as much as it does to medication? What if you get to co-create your own healing, rather than just waiting to be saved?

You don't have to fully believe in your new story yet. You just have to be curious enough to *crack the spine.*

## Reader Reflection:

1. **The Power of Choice and Belief in Healing:** Explore the profound connection between your thoughts, beliefs, and well-being. Find one belief about your

healing or life that feels disempowering. Write it down and reframe it as a positive affirmation. For example, transform "I can't heal from this" into "My body is capable of healing, and I trust the process."

2. **Tension Between Traditional and Holistic Approaches:** Do you wrestle with the possibility that a true solution may involve elements beyond conventional ideas? What tension do you experience when considering the rigidity of the norm and the fluid, empowering concepts of the mind-body connection?

3. **The Courage to Challenge Old Patterns:** The chapter reflects on the pressures of upbringing and how they contribute to health struggles, leading one to question long-held patterns. What familial or societal expectations have shaped your life? How do they impact your sense of self-worth or health? Are there old patterns you've outgrown but continue to hold onto? The body's suffering is a mask the mind holds up to hide what really suffers. What do you sense lies behind your symptoms?

4. **Radical Self-Love as an Approach to Healing:** The chapter emphasizes the transformative power of self-love through affirmations. The discovery that loving oneself can catalyze healing is both a challenge and an invitation. How do you currently practice self-love in your daily life? What could you add to deepen this practice? When you encounter resistance to the idea of self-love, where do you think it stems from?

## Affirmation:

*I embrace the power within me to heal.*

Scan the Code Below to View the Video for Chapter 23:
Or go to: https://youtu.be/u_1Yu1FcZSI

# Chapter 24

# Digging In The Dirt

**What You Bury, Your Body Remembers**
Vulnerability, emotional healing,
and the process of alchemizing past wounds.

*I honor the roots of my past
while allowing myself to grow beyond them.*

It felt like carrying a bowling ball up the stairs—in my stomach and my story.

Therapy wasn't new to me. But navigating it independently? That was. Therapy had been the other recommendation to come out of my court-ordered psych eval. I'd gone happily, hoping to be heard, knowing how dark my thoughts could be and how troubled our family was.

That help turned out to be short-lived.

Mom wanted a debriefing after every session. Even at fourteen, I knew they were a private affair—the therapist had said so. She interrogated me more. "I know you must talk about me."

I gazed longingly out my bedroom window, stalling and steeling myself against the invasion, marveling at the world outside. Maple trees burst into fiery autumn tones within their own cycles of change. I imagined the insides of other houses where kids didn't have to go to therapy—or if they did, got to keep it to themselves. It felt like my life wasn't mine, but tethered to my mother. Everything got filtered through her.

She laid her ace: "If you don't tell me what you talk about, then you can't go."

That was the end of therapy.

Even with the normalization of it within my degree and the referrals I made for clients in my job, it was still hard to admit that I couldn't get my mind right and needed help. I was hopeful for change, excited to see what I'd discover about myself, but also scared. What if I fell apart and couldn't pull myself together enough to handle Spanish class? What if my waterproof mascara wasn't up for the task?

What if we opened Pandora's Box and more spilled out than I could handle?

What if it made my Crohn's worse? Strong emotions triggered my symptoms. Crohn's, it seemed, didn't want me to be too upset or too happy; not too sad, but not too excited either. It wanted me to be flat-lined, more like Josh—easygoing and nonchalant. But oh, what a far cry I was from *that*.

I tried to blame Bitchisone for all my emotional instability and anger outbursts, but I knew that was just the gasoline. There were smoldering coals I couldn't tamp out, from a childhood that still burned.

Rounding the final corner in the hallway, I saw the open door to the therapist's office, and my breath fluttered into my lungs, forcing its way through a tightening rib cage, securing the periphery around my hesitant heart. Her office glowed warm. Her smile said, 'Your secrets are safe here.'

As the latch clicked, I felt the weight of my world shrink. For one hour, I belonged only to me and to my quest for greater self-awareness and acceptance. No one had to know. No one could stop me.

# GUT INSTINCTS

I sank into the cushy couch and exhaled so deeply it surprised me. I kicked off our conversation talking about Crohn's disease, how it got triggered when I got upset—"And I'm upset a lot." How I was failing all the treatments.

"Are *you* failing the treatments or are they failing you?" Her take turned the kaleidoscope ever so slightly, giving me a new picture.

"I'm doing everything right, but it's not enough." I told her about the drinking and drug use, how maybe Crohn's was *my* fault.

"You're very hard on yourself."

*Wow. She got that fast.* Her quick insight both concerned and encouraged me. I looked down at my toes, searching for the courage to revisit painful memories. I talked about my father leaving when I was four and my world breaking in half. How strict and controlling my mother was. "Anytime I expressed emotions, or got in a fight with my sister, or spilled my drink at a restaurant, I was told 'act your age.' But I was acting my age, so I looked to someone older and imitated them. Eventually feeling more like a little adult than a kid."

I sighed, surprised by the weight that memory held.

"Sounds like you had big responsibilities on your little shoulders." Her eyebrows raised and inched closer together out of concern. "Were you the oldest?"

I bristled. *And now we're at secrets.* Sweat sprouted from my armpits, sucking in my sleeves. As embarrassing as it was to talk about the specifics of my excrement, I almost preferred it to the chaotic composition of my family. *Do I say yes and leave out the part about my older brother? What do you call that? Oldest—sort of?*

I looked at the butterfly on the poster behind her, framing her head and telling the story 'just when the caterpillar though the world was over, it became a butterfly.' I loved butterflies.

Considered them the patron saints of transformation. *Maybe this office could be my cocoon.*

Realizing that confronting deep-seated emotional wounds was crucial to growth, I decided to state the truth.

She listened without flinching, her nods steady and eyes kind. Then she said something I didn't know I needed. "That's not a small thing. Of course it's shaped who you are."

"This disease is ripping me apart inside. I've started to explore some other, more esoteric approaches Do you know there are people out there beating cancer by dealing with their emotions?"

"That's amazing. It makes sense, though. Emotions are powerful energy you can't really escape. They find ways to express themselves." A legal pad balanced atop the draping of her flowery skirt

Within the sanctity of our sessions, I explored feelings that had never been fully expressed or processed. Being heard was so powerful, having someone's undivided attention so decadent. *No wonder I craved them as a child.* Sometimes, just listening to what I said would shift my perspective to a healthier and more accurate one.

Kind of like when I was a kid, afraid of monsters under the bed. Monsters—and monstrous thoughts—require dark and hidden places to exist. My approach was still childish—run as fast as I could and take a running jump to escape their evil talons.

Once daylight comes, the fear that monsters incite evaporates with the morning dew, seeming foolish. The glow of the floor lamp and my therapist's gentle processing became as powerful as the sun. We evaporated scary thought after scary thought.

Outside those appointments, I struggled to find the balance between vulnerability and resilience. My old thoughts kept coming back with the force of forbidden love.

"Have you tried journaling?" She asked.

"I used to when I was younger." I had a diary in a memory box kept under my bed with notes passed in class, keepsakes like movie stubs from *Footloose*—not being allowed to dance at that private school let me live vicariously through the rebellion playing out on the screen. And from Grease, seeing it transplanted the dream of my own transformation from an awkward and ostracized outcast to the cool, sexy Sandy, bringing boys to their knees.

My therapist nodded her recognition. "Yeah, I had something like that, too."

A shadow darkened the memory as a rogue wave of emotion rose and washed over me. My mother said she'd found my memory box while cleaning and, assuming it was garbage, threw it away. But she never cleaned my room; that was my job. "I was so mad and hurt, crying and yelling. She just blew it off as no big deal. It's silly now, but then, those things made me feel less alone because someone was feeling what I was feeling."

The therapist's mouth dropped open in surprise. "I don't see it as silly. She violated your boundaries."

My eyes watered, then wandered, landing on a framed print on a side table next to an aloe vera's plump strips—*Desiderata* telling me to go placidly among the noise.

*I thought it was 'walk tall and carry a big stick.'* I uncrossed and recrossed my legs. Little did I know, most of my healing journey would be about unlearning the survival patterns of self-protection that once kept me safe.

*Desiderata* answered: 'No less than the stars and the moon, you have a right to be here.'

*Wow.* Leaning back, I let the couch cushions, and words of my worth, enfold me.

I padded back down the brown carpet stairs, and it hit me how very far outside the comfort zone of self-preservation I was. *Is this really necessary?* I wondered.

The new voice in my head groaned. *How many more rats pressing levers and shock delivering experiments do you need???* I didn't know who this voice was. She sounded like me but wiser, more certain, and even-keeled. She did not waffle and she did not wonder.

She didn't apologize. She didn't explain.

She just knew.

And I was beginning to believe her.

By the time I ascended the cool, gray marbled stairs to my *Therapeutic Modalities: Practicum* class, we were both clear.

My body had sent up the bat signal and I couldn't unsee it.

If I wanted something different, I would have to do something different.

---

**Core Theme / Emotional Wound:** *No room of your own.* When your inner world gets invaded and your boundaries get violated, you learn to keep everything locked down—but what you bury doesn't disappear, it just finds another way to speak. This chapter confronts the trauma of *not being allowed to have a self, separate from others' needs or narratives.*

**Old Survival Pattern:** *Self-monitoring before self-knowing.* When you've learned to constantly edit yourself for safety, you lose track of what you actually think and feel beneath the surveillance. But healing means listening to yourself first, before checking if it's "allowed."

# GUT INSTINCTS

**Gut Instincts Healing Method Stage:** *Face*—the truth of your family dynamics, the impact of emotional repression, the monsters in the dark, and the grief in the light. This is the work of becoming the adult who listens to the child inside, and doesn't interrupt her.

**Reflection:**
I didn't realize it at the time, but that therapy office was the first space that truly belonged to *me*. Not the version filtered through my mother's lens. Not the girl who had to be easy, calm, in control. Just me—raw, unfiltered, unraveling in real time. And for once, I wasn't told to clean it up.

That room taught me that healing doesn't always look like doing. Sometimes it looks like *allowing.*

Allowing the tears.

Allowing the memories.

Allowing the truth to speak without needing to be justified.

Maybe you've learned to hold it all together, too. To keep your feelings zipped behind your ribs so no one gets uncomfortable. Maybe you've been the strong one for so long, you've forgotten what it feels like to just *be held.*

Strength isn't silence. And there's nothing weak about needing to be seen. There's wisdom in every tear you've swallowed. There's power in letting your story live in the light.

Maybe you, too, have always been the strong one. The responsible one. The one who kept the secrets and said the right things. The one who learned to tuck their feelings in so tight they stopped trying to speak.

But what if strength isn't stoicism? What if the bravest thing you can do is finally tell the truth—to someone safe, and then to yourself? This chapter invites you to view self-inquiry not as a fallback plan, but as a means of *reclamation.*

Of voice. Of softness. Of the parts of you that were never allowed to just be.

**Reader Reflection:**

1. **Safe Space Mapping.** Identify 1–2 people, spaces, or practices where you feel emotionally safe. Commit to spending more time there.
2. **Being Seen and Heard.** Have you experienced the power of being deeply listened to? What impact did it have? How can you create more moments of being heard, whether with friends, family, or professionals?
3. **Exploring Vulnerability.** Reflect on times when you needed to protect yourself emotionally—when have you pulled back from sharing and what led to that decision? Consider how you decide who to trust with your deepest emotions.
4. **Confronting Conditioning.** Reflect on your upbringing's impact on how you manage your emotions today. Are there family dynamics or beliefs that still influence your emotional habits? Has there been a moment when you realized you needed to shift those old ways?
5. **Stepping Outside Comfort Zones.** Think back to times you've stepped out of your comfort zone and experienced growth. What drove you to take that leap? How do you balance fear with the desire for change?

GUT INSTINCTS

## Affirmation:

*I have the courage to face my emotions, recalibrate my boundaries, and transform my wounds into wisdom.*

Scan the Code Below to View the Video for Chapter 24: Or go to: https://youtu.be/jbxVBoZ6bYU

## Chapter 25

# Changes

**Rewiring the Mind for Healing**
What you feed your mind is even more important
than what you feed your body.

*Today, I release my self-doubt and trust
in the transformative power of my thoughts.*

Included in the grant for my Parent Aide position was money for continued education. At a *Nurturing the Nurtures* conference, the keynote speaker illustrated the shift in social work from intervention to prevention with a parable. The gist was, rescuing clients in trouble demanded more effort and resources than figuring out the source of trouble and preventing it in the first place.

Additionally, preventive efforts were more cost-effective and easier to implement. 'A penny of prevention is worth a pound of cure.'

I could see how intervening between families and the courts could be prevented if we taught them the skills to be good parents in the first place.

Looking at my Crohn's, all I had were interventions. Food combining leaned into the prevention camp at least, but not far enough. Not when the medical mantra kept echoing: *We can't cure it because we don't know what causes it.*

One thought naturally and consistently followed: *If I knew what caused it, I could pull this weed out by the root.*

Steroids just snapped off the top, that's why it kept growing back.

I knew emotions drove my behavior. Therapy and journaling were helping me understand how emotions manifested in my body. My personal approach to prevention, I figured, would be identifying the source of the emotions.

Enter Jack Canfield.

As we attendees spilled out from the grand ballroom and into the hallway, I stumbled across something that would softly, yet majorly, shift the course of my life. A set of tapes titled *Self-Esteem and Peak Performance* pulled me over to a vendor's table like they were magnetized.

I had nothing in common with the pleated skirt and suit-wearing people on the cover wielding briefcases, but the word 'Self-Esteem' glowed like a beacon into the storm of my soul.

Despite all my advancements—job, grades, my resilience and resolve, pulling off a committed relationship with Josh—I still felt like shit about myself most of the time.

I bought the set of tapes without thinking, along with a daily affirmation book.

The next morning, I popped the first tape into my car stereo as I barreled down our gravel driveway for a home visit.

"I want you to try something," the clear and confident voice said. "Close your eyes."

*Okay, I obviously can't do that part. But go on...*

"You're on the roof of a very tall building. The city is quiet below you. You feel the wind. See the closeness of the clouds.

Now go to the edge. Put your toes up to it. Look down... see the cars so tiny below you."

He told us to open our eyes and asked how we felt. Gasps came through the speakers. "I'm sweating! My heart's pounding!"

*Me too—and my eyes were open!*

"Okay." Jack began again. "Close your eyes again. You're on the same tall building. But now, imagine you can fly. Maybe you have a jetpack. Maybe wings. Maybe you're a superhero."

That tweak greatly changed our reactions to joy, excitement, power.

"What changed?" Jack asked. "Same building. Same height. It was you... and the story you told yourself."

Dude had a point.

"When your mind changed, so did your experience."

Zzzt. Zzzzt. Zzzzt. I gripped the steering wheel while my brain short-circuited.

It wasn't the situation—it was the story.

He dropped more radical lines like breadcrumbs. "No matter what you say or do to me, I'm still a worthwhile person."

He said it with the confidence that came from naming the obvious. Like, worth wasn't earned. It just *was*.

I didn't believe it. But I tried saying it anyway, voice trembling. And I kept saying it, until it was vibrating in my chest.

The tapes went on heavy rotation, becoming an undeclared minor in *The Power of My Mind*.

Test anxiety got replaced with: *I know this stuff. I'm going to do well.* I turned in papers with: *I did my best,* instead of *I should've done better.* I let completed chapters feel like wins instead of skipping to the next to-do list item.

At night, I tallied my accomplishments instead of my failings.

## JENNIFER JUNIPER

One of Jack's stories really stuck with me. He didn't have the right ID to cash a check so the teller pushed it back. He slid it forward again and said, "I know, but this will work."

And it *did*.

His confidence wasn't cocky. It was quiet, grounded. Certain. I envied that. I practiced that. Telling my mind:

*I know, but this will work.*

*It's enough.*

*I'm enough.*

The affirmations in the book from the conference read like: *Things I Wish Were True.*

Still, I repeated them.

Even when my reflection mumbled, *Yeah right,* I said it anyway. Because for a moment, they felt better than the thoughts I'd inherited.

*Look at what a negative thought can do. Positive ones must be just as powerful.*

Bitchisone and affirmations fought like rivals. Some days I felt strong. Others, wobbly and spiraling. A forgotten fry order could ruin me. My body image was... brutal. Not only did I feel bad, but I *felt bad about my body.* Exercise didn't work. My hunger was ferocious. Jeans kept getting tighter. The steroidal scream drowning out every effort.

But the affirmations? They were like soft override switches. Each one, a subtle reframe.

I saw them work in my clients as well. Watching them shift—hearing new words emerge where shame used to live—cheered me on.

Patterns could be disrupted.

Trauma didn't get the last word.

Belief could be restructured.

*Today, I value peace over perfection.*

Another total reversal of thought that *felt* right.

## GUT INSTINCTS

All that driving gave me time to process. Affirmations were like easy-to-digest fruit. My childhood conditioning? A heap of poorly combined leftovers. Therapy and journaling sorted and separated, turning it over until it became soul compost helping something new grow.

It took just a glimmer of a new belief to see that peace was possible. When I got an A- on a paper, a fresh voice whispered: *Still an A. You worked hard on that.*

It felt as foreign as Spanish class, but I kept practicing.

*Come what may, I am healing.*

I didn't know how true that one was. But I knew this—every new thought, every morning mantra, every gentle override was a step in the right direction.

\*\*\*

There is only one picture of my college graduation. I didn't want any, but my friend's mom insisted.

"You'll regret it!" she bubbled, snapping the photo.

My head looks like a bowling ball balanced between cap and gown—moon face, they called it—a side effect of steroids. I'm sporting a double chin. I am not smiling.

I'd graduated with honors. Had a job in my field. And still, a realization echoed louder than any applause—the medicine wasn't working. The sulfa drugs didn't seem to help at all, and the steroids only helped while I was on them—and I couldn't stay on them.

The look on my face said everything: a woman at the end of her schooling, *and* her rope.

**Core Theme / Emotional Wound:** *Unworthiness + mental self-punishment.* This chapter shines a spotlight on the ways internal narratives keep us sick, small, and spiraling. The wound here is a fundamental *doubt of worthiness*, paired with the pressure to always "do better."

**Old Survival Pattern:** *Internalized shame.* You can trace how you weaponize your thoughts against yourself. "I'm failing." "It's my fault." "I'm not enough." We start to notice and *challenge* those loops.

**Gut Instincts Healing Stage:** *Filter → Follow.* This is the pivot chapter—*filtering* out the old story *(I'm the problem, something's wrong with me. I need fixing)* and beginning to *follow* a new one *(I have wisdom worth listening to. Maybe I can trust myself on this).*

**Reflection:**
Back then, I didn't know affirmations could be more than wishful thinking. I just knew the thoughts I *had* weren't helping I didn't believe any of them were true at first. But something in me wanted to, and that was enough.

So I listened. I repeated. I practiced a new way of thinking before I believed it. Sometimes, that's what true change asks of us—to speak the truth before we fully trust it.

Maybe you've done everything "right" and still feel like it's never enough. Perhaps your inner voice is harsher than any doctor you've met. Maybe you've been trained to motivate yourself with shame, and wonder why you still feel stuck.

But what if love works better? What if self-worth isn't something you earn—but something you *reclaim*?

And what if the most radical healing isn't just shifting your symptoms, but changing the way you speak to yourself when no one else can hear?

**Reader Reflection:**

1. **The Power of Perspective.** Can you identify ways your thoughts have held you back, like the rooftop scenario? How have limiting beliefs or fears shaped your decisions? Have you ever held yourself back simply because you feared failure, even in a seemingly safe situation?
2. **The Influence of Self-Talk.** How often do you use affirmations or positive self-talk? What does your inner voice usually sound like? Consider the narrative you often hear in your mind—do you focus on what's going wrong, or can you begin to see the opportunity for growth even in challenges?
3. **Claiming Your Growth.** What transformations in your life are you proud of, but might not celebrate enough? Reflect on the changes in your life that you've worked hard for but might downplay because we don't meet your "perfectionist" standards. Acknowledge these quietly celebrated achievements.
4. **Letting Peace Lead.** How would your life look if you chose peace over performance? Consider one area of your life where you typically strive for perfection. What would happen if you let unconditional self-love and acceptance take the place of relentless striving?

JENNIFER JUNIPER

## Affirmation:

*I dare to face my emotions, recalibrate my boundaries, and transform my wounds into wisdom.*

Scan the Code Below to View the Video for Chapter 25: Or go to: https://youtu.be/V0dS7rz9Y0c

## Chapter 26

# Runnin' Down A Dream

### From Seeking Answers to Trusting Instincts
Finding your way by following what resonates.

*I am a possibility, and my journey is a canvas where healing and growth unfold with every brushstroke I make.*

Technically, I hadn't graduated. Those pesky Spanish credits still lingered. Foreign language classes met four days a week, but time-wise and gas money-wise, I had to limit my schedule to three. Getting my degree meant stacking classes Tetris-style and learning Spanish as a self-study—the worst way to learn a language. I stalled out on taking the final exam because I knew it would ding my GPA.

But I wouldn't let that tiny, insignificant detail stop me from chasing my dream job.

The position of Prevention/Intervention Specialist was a perfect fit, so I applied and got the interview. Sitting at the end of a shiny, long, mahogany table, facing a man with salt-and-pepper hair—swiveled sideways with legs crossed, as men in power often do—I was equal parts intimidated and determined. At the end, when he asked if I had anything to add, I didn't hesitate. "Yes. I think you should hire me. I'm perfect for this job, and whatever I don't know, I can learn."

## JENNIFER JUNIPER

Walking to my car, I felt a sense of pride that determination had edged out the intimidation. I calculated that there would be enough time to get my diploma before HR requested it. *It's a long shot anyway.*

\*\*\*

"Welcome," said the executive director—swiveled-sideways guy—leaning against the doorframe of my new office. "And congratulations!"

"Thank you." I replied with a smile, still trying to get comfortable with the new chair, still trying to believe I'd actually gotten the job.

"Did you know you beat out a stack of applicants this thick?" He held up his fingers two inches apart. "Some had master's degrees and were internal transfers."

"No," I answered, wide-eyed. *Good thing. I'd been nervous enough.*

"Do you know why I hired you?" he asked, smiling.

Still in shock, I could only shake my head.

"I asked everyone the same question at the end—whether they had anything to add. You were the only one that did."

Passion and determination had seemed like a good way to beef up my skimpy resume, and I was passionate. He'd seen a confident woman asserting herself. Looking through his eyes, I caught a glimpse of her, too.

One of those transfer requests had been from an alcohol and drug abuse counselor. She told me when we partnered for a project: a deferred prosecution program educating DUI first offenders on alcoholism. In her part of the presentation, Robin illustrated the roles people play in an alcoholic home families by drawing a diagram of dysfunction.

The more she drew, the more I made sense.

## GUT INSTINCTS

The Hero—their job it was to raise the family's esteem—only received attention for achievements, leaving their inner needs unmet.

Scapegoat also rang true—the lightning rod for pain and stress. The one who goes against the rules, and in doing so, sometimes brings help to the family. (I'd tried.)

I also learned *(who's this class for, anyway!?)* that when you start using, you stop growing emotionally. Going under the bleachers at football games—and all the other ways I'd tried to escape the pain of growing up in my chaotic family—hadn't gotten me out of those awkward developmental lessons. They only arrested my development and kicked my curriculum down the road.

The more she talked, the wider my lens zoomed out. Healing was more than physical. It required unearthing the roots of my emotional pain and psychological dysfunction.

Robin may have started out as a reluctant partner, but the shared vulnerability of our similar health struggles soon created a bond. When my face ballooned from another round of steroids, she asked about it knowingly, and confided her own diagnosis of ulcerative colitis. Her confession felt like a lifeline. I'd finally found a comrade in this silent army, marching in the same fatigues.

But learning about her colostomy bag was bittersweet. Ulcerative colitis was a sister disease to Crohn's, but since it affected the colon only, it had an endgame—removing it. Mine did not. Crohn's traveled farther. I had it throughout my entire digestive system, from entrance to exit.

So while I got the position, she got the cure.

"You don't have to go it alone," Robin offered one particularly rough day. "There's a Crohn's & Colitis Foundation—you can write them for resources. There's even a support group at the hospital."

## JENNIFER JUNIPER

. . .

Sterility's stinging smell greeted me once again, following my descent into the basement, down a hallway of stark white walls made gray by buzzing fluorescent lights. My nerves buzzed with them.

I envisioned empathetic nods, shared strategies, glimmers of hope. Camaraderie. Hugs, maybe. I settled best I could into a cold, metal folding chair, nestling into the circle like a huddle for community and insights. *Okay, let's figure this out!*

As person after person lamented their treatment, their doctors, their bowels, their parents, their partners, their very existence, my hopeful smile faded. A lively debate ensued over the best flavors of meal replacement drinks, dimming my inner light of positivity and possibility.

One woman's husband posted a list of "safe foods" on the fridge and blamed her for flares when she deviated. Another waitress wore a diaper at work. Many were on disability, unable to hold jobs. All had resigned themselves to this being their lot.

There was no succor in the circle. Hope had vacated and left no forwarding address.

We all had the same disease, but we were handling it in very different ways. If I stayed, I feared I'd slowly deflate my dream of thriving down to merely surviving—which wasn't an option.

I climbed the stairs and vowed never to return. *I'll die if I hang here with them.*

The next morning, Saturday, with no work and Josh still sleeping, I made a second cup of coffee and grabbed the thick resource guide from the Crohn's & Colitis Foundation. I didn't just read it—I mined it. Skipping what I already knew, I landed on the last chapter: *Surgery*.

The mother lode.

The more I read about bowel resections, the more excited I got. Cutting out the bad and sewing up the good sounded like my ticket off such a crazy ride. I grabbed my new insurance card and set out to find someone to cut me open.

While waiting for the consult, I hit the books.

Encouraged by *Love, Medicine & Miracles*, I dove deeper. Dr. Siegel continued. "I wanted to make people aware they were not statistics or probabilities, but possibilities..."

*I'm a possibility*. I let that reframe do its magic.

He spoke of intuitive knowledge—wisdom not available to the intellect. Yes. My gut instincts were guiding me all along—to my major, my school, at those job interviews, in choosing the second group, sticking with proper food combining even when my doctor doubted.

Of course. *Nobody knows my body like I do.* Doctors could advise, *but I'm the one living with it.*

He referenced a study. Women with advanced breast cancer who received group therapy and autohypnosis doubled their survival time compared to those receiving traditional treatment alone. Those women and their results told me I was on the right track. *Keep going, keep looking, keep dealing with the pain of the past.*

Therapy and journaling were the one-two punch of processing all those past losses. That thread of childhood trauma and its manifestations wove itself through my personal health history, my clients' progress, my education, and confirmed further by these women's successes.

I didn't have it in me to be a passive patient. I was becoming my own healer. Not my doctors. Not the pills. Not my boyfriend. No one else could save me but me.

Then came another Siegel gem: 'I want to add self-healing to your options.'

I liked the sound of that. But... *how?*

A quote from Franz Alexander, M.D. answered. 'The mind rules the body. It's the most fundamental fact we know about life.'

I read it again. *My mind rules my body?*

It felt like the opposite. My body consumed my thoughts, especially on bad days. But I wanted it to be true. *Needed* it to be true.

Dr. Siegel served up more sage wisdom. Disease can be used to heal a life.'

That echoed Louise Hay. I reached for *You Can Heal Your Life* and plunged into the cherry-red center of the rainbow-radiating heart on its cover, like the Starship Enterprise into a wormhole.

'Even self-hatred is only hating a thought you have about yourself. Change the thought, and the feeling must go.'

*It can't be that easy.* But then I remembered the rooftop from those Canfield tapes. 'It wasn't the building that changed. I was your belief about the building.' It all converged into a brighter and brighter beam in the darkness.

Healing wasn't some far-off miracle. It was a possibility rooted in action. My journals became a haven. Each insight added a tool to my growing kit.

Maybe I hadn't just picked a psych major randomly. Perhaps I'd been preparing for this all along.

Louise answered. *I listen with love to my body's messages.*

Was my body trying to tell me something?

As I closed the book, I realized that healing wasn't about fixing my broken bits. It was about extracting the wisdom from the cracks. For the first time, I wasn't just running from my disease. I was running toward something greater—my wholeness.

I didn't have all the answers. But at least I had a compass.

---

**Core Theme / Emotional Wound:** *The ache of almost belonging.* You enter systems looking for solidarity—medical, professional, personal relationships—where offers are partial but never full recognition. You're left carrying the burden of forging your own path while everyone else follows the map.

**Old Survival Pattern:** *Seeking external validation for internal knowing.* You've learned to look outward first—to experts, credentials, established programs—for permission to trust what you already sense is true. But growth means recognizing when nothing external reflects your truth, the answer isn't to doubt yourself—it's to trust yourself more.

**Gut Instincts Stage:** *Follow + Filter.* Choosing what resonates and releasing what doesn't. You're learning to trust your inner "yes" over external authority, filtering out voices of limitation, and following the trail of what actually moves you forward— even when you're the only one on the path.

**Reflection:**
Looking back now, I realize I didn't just want solutions—I wanted resonance. I didn't need people to fix me. I needed someone to say, "Me too," without collapsing into defeat.

I vowed never to return to that support group, not because I knew what healing looked like, but because I knew it didn't look like that.

If you've ever walked into a room hoping to feel seen— and left more invisible than when you entered—you know this ache. And you know this truth: not every group is your group. Not every expert is your guide. Not every path gives you power.

But maybe what's real is this: your intuition never left. It's still here. Quietly guiding. Waiting for you to run, not away from your pain, but toward the possibility of something more

**Reader Reflection:**

1. **Trusting Your Instincts.** Take a moment to think about times in your life when your instincts nudged you toward a decision, even if it seemed unconventional or uncertain. What did it feel like to trust that inner voice? Were there moments when you ignored it, and how did those situations turn out?

    Reflect on how those experiences have shaped your ability to tune in to your intuition. Where in your life are you currently hesitating to trust your instincts? Are you second-guessing yourself because of fear, external opinions, or uncertainty?

2. **Healing as a Journey.** How does the idea of healing as a continuous, evolving journey resonate with you? Reflect on how your understanding of healing has evolved over time. Have you noticed any shifts in how you view your body, your emotions, or life experiences?

3. **Challenging the Narrative.** Reflect on any stories you've been telling yourself about your limitations, health, or past experiences. How might those stories be holding you back from your potential? What new

narrative can you create to open up possibilities for growth and healing?

4. **The Power of Words and Beliefs.** How do your thoughts and beliefs influence your current healing journey? What empowering beliefs about yourself and your health can you begin to adopt to encourage healing and transformation?

## Affirmation:

*I trust my inner wisdom to guide me.
My instincts serve as the compass that guides me toward healing, truth, and alignment with my best self.*

Scan the Code Below to View the Video for Chapter 26:
Or go to: https://youtu.be/KH2vLOfyTY8

## Chapter 27

# The Sound of Silence

### Your Center in the Storm
The stillness you cultivate in calm becomes your anchor in chaos.

*I create peace within myself,
and that peace radiates outward,
grounding me through life's challenges.*

With a new job and a new car (one without rust and a check engine light), Josh and I began shopping for a new home. Life was expanding in all directions, like I'd arrived on some new precipice of adulthood.

Of all the parts of the job I was drawn to, the role of lead facilitator for *The Nurturing Program for Families of Adolescents* excited me most. An immersive, twelve-week program addressing the entire family system, it aimed to replace abusive behaviors with nurturing ones by building parents' self-worth, empathy, and fostering bonding and attachment.

The theory was revolutionary: the "problem child" was seen as the barometer of the family's dysfunction. Their disobedience was a distress signal.

Each week we used discussions, role-play, expressive arts, and assessments to facilitate healthier parent-child interactions. Watching families healing together, I couldn't help but wonder how different things might've been for my own family. But we never sought help.

Every session closed with a guided meditation. I volunteered to read the first one. Another facilitator dimmed the lights while everyone got comfortable lying on the floor.

My voice started steady but uncertain, like the first drop of rain before a summer storm. My breathing slowed. I noticed my shoulders softening. Even my belly, clenched so tightly for so long, began to unfurl.

Franz was right. My mind *did rule* my body.

If affirmations put me back in the driver's seat with my mind, meditation slowed my speed. A winning combination for a Tasmanian Devil used to ricocheting off of everything. I stopped bracing, started breathing. At every red light or any of life's pauses, I relaxed into stillness. My fingertips tingled, and I created a harmonizing hum beneath my skin.

Bathrooms turned into a type of sanctuary. In the span of five breaths, I felt my nervous system reset. Hungry for more, I ordered a meditation tape from the back of *You Can Heal Your Life*.

Meditation became my traveling sanctuary, revealing a kind of control I'd never known over my inner world. My emotional eruptions began to cool. The anxiety that churned in my gut loosened its grip. It wasn't just relaxation—it was restoration. Each conscious breath stitching together fractured parts of me, creating a calm I didn't know was possible.

That feeling came to life inside the home of one of my co-facilitators. Dawn's place looked, smelled, and felt like everything I was learning and becoming. Spiritual, not religious, and filled with weathered wood, soft light, a Buddha fountain at the door, with the *Serenity Prayer* hanging framed on the wall. Candles glowed in the bathroom, next to books that mirrored my growing collection.

The Zen was palpable.

Dawn had been through her own storms. She was breaking the cycle of abuse she'd grown up with. And while I resonated with her grit, I envied her gentleness. A magic carpet of trust seemed to glide beneath her feet. She was confident but calm. Determined but soft. The embodiment of grace. Her whole family was, even the kids.

Josh, by contrast, didn't meet me in these places. He nodded when I shared metaphysical insights or book passages, but I could tell he didn't understand. He never volleyed anything back. His humor and even keel continued their balance of my liveliness, but when it came to my deeper explorations, I was journeying alone.

### Hello, darkness, my old friend

My dad's death unmoored me.

Found in bed, alone, in a diabetic coma—he'd left me for the last time. My first thought was the same as all the other times—*I wish it were my mother instead.* The tether between Dad and me could stretch amazingly—and uncomfortably—far, but we always had some connection, no matter how taut. If I pulled and pulled and pulled, eventually, he'd come back to me.

I guessed it finally snapped in the storm of his soul. Leaving me untethered.

I imagined his last moments on repeat. Was the insulin too far away? Or just too hard to reach for one more time? Dad always did gamble with his diabetes. Was it Russian roulette?

Grief flooded in, fast and wide. I was twenty-two. Too young to bury my father. The link to my identity severed, again. Permanently this time. I would forever be a Daddy's Girl without a daddy.

His being single and my being the oldest (kind of) made me the executor of the estate. My burden was different. Heavier. My sister hung with our mom in the wings of another scene. Even my grandpa didn't get it. I stood toe-to-toe with my dad's Dad, arguing over what to bury him in.

"A suit and tie," Grandpa said. "It's tradition."

"He'd hate that." I barked back. "He doesn't even own one!"

His favorite shirt—the one he wore the most and embarrassed me the most—was a garish Hawaiian shirt in flaming sunset colors. He'd wear that.

I'd felt voiceless in the family for so long, swept along by the choices and expectations of others. But in that moment, I stood my ground, not just for his legacy but for the version of myself who believed in honoring what truly matters.

Planning the service was another battle. Grandpa wanted a Catholic priest. But Dad wasn't Catholic—far from it with his crystals, psychic fairs, and library of enlightenment. He didn't have a dogmatic bone in his body.

I agreed to *Amazing Grace* because I loved it and it always brought me comfort. But the rest of the playlist? That needed to reflect Dad's tastes. If this was the last time those who loved him would see him, we needed to recognize him and remember his essence.

The funeral preparations broke whatever bond remained between my mother and me. Every tear I shed defined as betrayal. "It's like you loved him more than me."

*Can't I even grieve in peace?*

Adding to the list of what I couldn't deal with was the radio static of knowing I wasn't the eldest child. Executor of the estate was my brother Mark's job. The one I barely knew about and couldn't ask about—a mystery within an enigma.

Grief stacked on grief.

## GUT INSTINCTS

Before the viewing, Uncle Denny walked between my sister and me, one arm around each of us, toward the casket. I felt the smooth, cool polyester of his dark suit, his arm flexing, his grip tightening under my ribcage to catch me as my knees buckled.

My body said what my mouth couldn't. *This weight is too heavy for me.*

---

**Core Theme / Emotional Wound:** *Holding it together when everything's falling apart.* Being the "strong one" means your grief gets postponed, your needs get minimized, and your breaking point becomes everyone else's inconvenience.

**Old Survival Pattern:** *Silent competence over authentic expression.* Better to be the reliable one who keeps it together than the messy one whose grief makes others uncomfortable—even when the silence cost you your relationship with yourself.

**Gut Instincts Method Stage:** — *Face + Follow.* Honoring the grief process, along with what remains unsaid and was never healed. Fighting for what feels right in the face of resistance.

We are also starting to acknowledge that healing doesn't just require knowing the truth—it requires making space for it.

**Reflection:**
I didn't just lose my father—I lost the version of myself who believed he'd always come back. When the silence fell for good, something else rose in me. Not just grief, but clarity. A call to protect my peace. To build a life where I didn't have to guess if love was coming back.

Maybe you've felt that too—the ache of unfinished conversations, the haunting silence of someone who never fully arrived, or left too soon. Loss doesn't always come with closure. But it can bring clarity.

You don't need permission to grieve someone who wasn't all there to begin with. What if the peace you crave doesn't come from resolution, but from choosing yourself, anyway?

**Reader Reflection:**

1. **Meditation as Healing.** Think about a time when you felt overwhelmed or lost in the chaos of life. How might pausing to breathe and reflect have shifted your perspective? Reflect on a moment when intentional stillness brought clarity or relief. What can you do to make mindfulness a more regular part of your day?
2. **Relationships and Spiritual Growth.** Consider how family roles and unresolved tensions shape your emotional landscape. Are there patterns you want to shift? How can you cultivate relationships that align with your inner growth?
3. **Grief as a Teacher.** Loss is one of life's most difficult experiences, but it often reveals what matters most. Reflect on a loss in your life. What lessons or strengths have come from it? How has it shaped your journey?

## Affirmation:

*My peace is built through self-trust.
I am free to say all I need to say,
to fully grieve for as long as necessary.*

Scan the Code Below to View the Video for Chapter 27:
Or go to: https://youtu.be/UTmktTdJasY

# Chapter 28

# Don't Give Up

### Rewriting the Rules
When there's no way forward, you have to make one.

*I swallowed the dice; I make my own luck now.*
~Dessa

The doctor's tie was a fish. The coffee cup on his desk, a fish—tail flipped up, forming a handle. *Guess the man likes to fish on his days off from cutting into people.* A joke was swimming around in there somewhere, scalpels. . . scaling, but Bitch-isone had stolen my sense of humor—along with my regular-sized clothes and my appetite's off-switch—and I didn't feel much like chit-chatting.

I was there for one, sole, serious purpose.

"You're not a candidate for surgery," the doctor said as he slammed the door of my file shut, clasping his hands on top of it for emphasis. His smile conveyed that he was satisfied that all he needed to know about my insides was inside.

I smiled back, then scanned the room. Stalling. Searching for some clue about this Fish Doctor. There was a picture of his wife on his desk. She seemed nice. Pretty. *She probably bought him that mug and tie for.* . . my eyes landed on the other framed photos—*Father's Day.*

But I was tired of being polite and compliant with every test ordered and prescription scribbled on a pad. Tired of the false hope the pharmacy offered, tired of choking on horse-sized pellets of promise. Sick of their side effects. Sick of doctors pushing their fingers into the places that hurt and asking, 'Does this hurt?'

I'd done everything asked of me, to a T.

Only to end up in the ER.

Again.

Getting blood sucked out of one vein while bags of IV fluid and steroids emptied into another—veins that curled up and hid every time a needle got near. 'Milkshakes' of sludge, watching my digestive system glow alive on a monitor above my bed (which was only cool the first few times), only to leave with the same pills and the same plan.

My chest tightened. My throat ached and swelled. I blinked back the surge filling my eyes, spilling their salty streams instead. "I don't know what else to do," I croaked. "I've tried *everything*."

Casting about, I detailed the impossible cycle of steroids: the weight gain, the temper, insomnia, then flare-ups when I weaned off, and the trips to the emergency room in the middle of the night to get pumped full of more. I name-dropped case studies, cited stats, pitched bowel resections like miracle cures—hoping to reel him in.

I was still eyeing surgery as my escape hatch—my chance to get off the medical merry-go-round, even for a minute.

"Please." I leaned forward, into the promise this option held, desperation creeping into my voice. "I think this will work. I *need* it to."

He softened, tipping his head to one side, nodding along with my soliloquy in empathy. "Look. You have this disease everywhere," motioning to my file for backup, "I can't take it all out, or you'll have even worse problems."

I looked past him to the framed degrees on his wall, the bookcase they flanked. *He probably thinks they've told him everything he needs to know about Crohn's Disease. But they haven't told him about me.* He didn't know how I'd mastered deep breathing to the point of making my fingers and toes tingle with relaxation, how I got in mini-meditations at red lights. Or that I read every healing story I could get my hands on.

*There's more to me than what's in my file.*

I squinted. Was *Love, Medicine & Miracles* in that bookcase? Maybe he's never even heard of You Can Heal Your Life.

But the biggest, most important thing he didn't know was that I had chosen the *second* group.

His rejection of the only treatment option I had left, piled on top of years of being confronted with the direness of my condition, triggered tears. The dashing of my dream to overcome my disease made them flow harder. I thought I would breeze in, get acquainted, open my calendar, and we'd set a date.

"I'm so sorry," he sounded sincere, "But these people that you read about, they don't have it like you do."

My mind abandoned its resolve and flashed back to the hospital, the coloring page illustrating my diagnosis; all those dashes. It was bad. The Fish Doc was right.

I rode in on a wave of confidence in this resolution and crashed, smashed against the rocks of reality. His words washed into me, drowning my hope. Gutted, I sank back into my chair, a cushiony velour with a scalloped curved back, belonging more to a living room than a doctor's office. Perhaps to serve as soft support while cutting and carving was discussed.

My mind rewound to Dr. Cute & Confident, back to the two groups. *I want the second group, dammit! I claimed it. And these people with the stethoscopes aren't getting me there.*

Every cell in my body shook its head no, until my insides whirlpooled. A flood of disappointment threatened to capsize, making me reach for anything that floated. The books, tapes, healing stories, the courage to stand up for a funeral that reflected my father, that line from The Little Prince—*one sees clearly only with the heart. Anything essential is invisible to the eyes.*

Maybe it was the affirmations empowering me and the meditations centering me.

Maybe I was desperate.

I couldn't keep shuffling the deck and hoping for a better hand. I needed a game-changer. I was done playing defense with this disease. I thirsted for a crack at offense.

Maybe if he had on a different tie and wasn't gripping a porcelain tail.

My heart abducted my mind, and with steady certainty said. "I'm not leaving until you agree to operate."

The words spilled from somewhere deeper than just frustration, pooling around our feet and shocking us both. *Maybe freedom really is just another word for nothing left to lose.* I was already sick and suffering with no lasting relief in sight.

In that, my boldest of bold moments, I realized something. I didn't need approval. I didn't need anyone to validate my right to heal. The decision wasn't in their hands anymore. It was in mine.

Fish Doc sighed emphatically. "Look, even if I took out the worst part, you'd only get about six months of remission. And then it would come back, probably right where I sewed you back together."

## GUT INSTINCTS

"SIX MONTHS!?" The mere possibility propelled me to the edge of my seat. *Six months?!* My brain savored the very thought of it. It sounded like an eternity. "I'll take it! I can't even get a few weeks! And at least I'll get a chance at a fresh start, instead of being behind the eight ball all the time!"

Shock registered across his face as I used the justification for rejection to help make my case. He took a slow sip from his fish mug.

*Poor guy. Probably thought this would be an open-and-shut case, and he'd get to go to lunch early.*

"You know, it's usually me trying to convince people to have surgery, not the other way around." Then he opened his calendar. "Looks like my next opening is in two weeks."

I had him.

Hook,

line,

and

sinker.

"That's too soon." My decision was instant. The Nurturing Program was in the sweet spot, where real change was taking root—patterns breaking, trust building, families transforming. Leaving now would be like bailing on a symphony halfway through its crescendo.

I couldn't abandon the families or their transformations— work that had kept me grounded and balanced while my body betrayed me, shining a beacon of hope into my personal transformation. If I were going to squeeze every bit out of the 'six months, tops' remission time, I needed all the help like that I could get.

*I've been miserable for years. What's a couple more weeks?*

Confusion crossed his face, followed by exasperation and, finally, resignation. He smoothed his fish tie and sighed. "When does it finish?"

I rose and shook his hand, gushing gratitude and babbling, "You won't regret it, doc."

The look on his face said he wasn't entirely convinced. But I didn't care. I just needed him to do it. I'd take it from there.

---

**Core Theme / Emotional Wound:** *Invalidation + Powerlessness.* You've done everything "right"—played by the rules, followed the protocols, swallowed every promise, and still been dismissed. This chapter crystallizes the wound of not being seen *even at your breaking point*—and the deeper grief of gatekeeping. It's not just your health on the line—it's your agency.

**Old Survival Pattern:** *Deference → Defiance.* The unconscious pattern here is over-compliance, learned from a lifetime of needing approval to feel safe. You've been "the good patient" (or partner, parent, employee) until now. This chapter marks the *rupture* of that pattern and the rise of your refusal to be told what you're allowed to hope for.

**Gut Instincts Healing Method Stage:** *Follow.* You're no longer seeking validation. You're following your inner knowing. The power dynamic flips here—you are the one with clarity, not the credentials. What do you choose to believe? This is your turning point: intuitive rebellion with purpose.

**Reflection:**
I wasn't begging for surgery. I was claiming my right to hope. So many of us were taught to defer, to doubt ourselves, to believe that an expert knows what we need better than we do.

Sometimes healing begins not with agreement, but with refusal. You don't need permission to want more. You don't have to wait for approval to pursue what feels true. What if your fiercest moment of life is the one that sets you free?

**Reader Reflection:**

1. **Advocating for Yourself in Difficult Situations.** Think about a time when you had to challenge an authority figure or push back against a decision. What emotions came up for you, and how did you navigate them?
2. **Finding Strength in Resistance.** Reflect on moments when you faced resistance—whether from others or within yourself. How did you move forward despite it? What helped you stay anchored in your truth?
3. **Trusting Your Inner Compass.** Are there moments in your life when you trusted your instincts even when others doubted you? How did following your inner guidance change the outcome?
4. **Reevaluating Traditional Authority.** How do you determine when to trust professionals or experts and when to question their recommendations? What role does intuition play in those decisions?
5. **Personal Growth Through Professional Work.** Think about how your work or passions have helped you grow as a person. What lessons have you learned from helping others that you now apply to yourself?

JENNIFER JUNIPER

## Affirmation:

*I am the ultimate authority on my life and my healing.
I trust myself to make decisions
that align with my highest good.*

Scan the Code Below to View the Video for Chapter 28:
Or go to: https://youtu.be/9YxKw7NgsE0

# Chapter 29

# This Woman's Work

### The Mind as Medicine
Integration, complete ownership, and advocacy.

*"Can you promise that I will come back?"*
*Asked Bilbo Baggins*
*"No." Answered Gandalf.*
*"And if you do, you'll not be the same."*
*~The Hobbit: An Unexpected Journey*

It was a bitchy, bursting-at-the-seams six weeks, brimming with hope. I could stay on full-dose steroids, no numbers plotted on the calendar tapering me off, no threat of a flare-up turning my world upside down, no worry of Josh's and my sleep being interrupted by a mad midnight dash to the ER. No worry about the weight gain or the moonface—surgery would fix it all.

I had the scaffolding; it was time to build another floor. I needed to level up the mind-body connection so I could milk every second out of my six-month remission.

Taking out the worst and sewing the better parts back together sounded a lot like what we did in therapy. I locked our conversations in an inner vault and sprung the lock when

I got a quiet moment for introspection—like late at night when the steroids made it hard to sleep.

I crossed the living room, lace curtains casting moon shine cutouts on the carpet. Something I'd said about being hardwired for loss was replaying. 'I thought the world was my oyster, but maybe it's more like my castle. Complete with moat and palace guards.'

'Interesting...' My therapist liked to coo that word, giving hang time to the latest lob from my subconscious. Then she'd expand on it. 'Having a chronic illness is a kind of grief. The loss of your body's proper functioning. Loss of a normal life. Loss of belonging.'

Loss was something I needed to process, not mitigate—I wasn't an insurance company. *Deal with my feelings* and *If they beat cancer, I can beat Crohn's* were two drumsticks whittled from Love, *Medicine & Miracles* beating against my heart. The rhythm I marched to when approaching my therapist's door to psyche myself up to pull another well-taped cardboard box from. In one of those boxes were all the reasons I felt unworthy.

Basements are scary. Better to have someone hold the flashlight—and your hand.

One of those boxes was my self-worth. No matter how hard I strived to earn my self-worth, it remained just out of reach. Each accomplishment only seemed to reset it, every accolade evaporated as soon as the person stopped delivering it. I was good at things, but I just didn't feel like *I* was good.

Not good enough anyway.

On my therapist's couch, I nodded along with 'Worth isn't earned but inherent in our very being,' secure in a more solid sense of myself. Getting good grades, doing a good job, being liked, those were things I *did*, not who I was. *Separate doing from being, got it.*

But when I got around other people, I couldn't get comfortable. I scanned any room I entered—first, to lock in a bathroom location and second, to figure out who to be.

'Like a chameleon,' said my therapist.

'Like a contortionist,' I countered.

'A sense of belonging is the opposite of trying to fit in. You deserve to be in every room you enter.'

I carried her words with me—and if push came to shove, even acted like they were true—but eventually I'd revert to a little girl hoping to get picked for the kickball team. I hated it.

If negative self-talk meant continuing to drink the poisonous messaging of my past, then affirmations were the elixir. I canceled out any damaging ones with *I'm not available for that thought.* Or I'd repeat the self-condemning thought, putting '*I used to*' before it.

From *I'm always late* to *I used to always be late.*

*I used to be so clumsy.*

*I used to have no idea what my body needs.*

"I used to" reset my future by unhitching it from the past.

Slowly, with lots of repetition and dedication, I started to gain the self-worth I'd been seeking my entire life.

I settled in next to my inheritance—Dad's massive music collection. Thumbing through the CDs, I searched for instrumentals to enhance the meditations at the end of the Nurturing Program sessions. Dad naming me after a song must've triggered the need for a soundtrack. From a young age, I knew music's power—its ability to match any mood, to soothe, give words to my soul, read my mind.

'Michael was like a firecracker spinning and sparking on the sidewalk on Fourth of July—dazzling and vivid. But as you watch, captivated by its brilliance, you think, *this can't last.*'

## JENNIFER JUNIPER

I couldn't think of a more accurate metaphor.

I settled in next to my inheritance—Dad's massive music collection. Thumbing through the CDs, I searched for instrumentals to enhance the meditations at the end of the Nurturing Program sessions. Dad naming me after a song must've triggered the need for a soundtrack to my life. From a young age, I knew music's power—its ability to match any mood, to soothe, give words to my soul, open my mind.

*God he loved music.*

Walking into Dad's living room was like entering a DJ booth. His ever-increasing collection pushed the sofa out until it was in the dining room, yet he could extract any album from anywhere, in any genre, in seconds.

Grief put a dimmer switch on my world.

A fellow columnist from the newspaper where dad worked delivered the eulogy. I'm not sure how that came to be—did he make some sincere offer of 'let me know if there's anything I can do,' and I said, 'How about the eulogy?' He saw my dad almost every day for decades and had a way with words—I was a big fan of his weekly column.

There I was, carrying on his legacy with a jewel case open in my lap and a Sharpie in hand, ready to mark the best tracks with a black dot.

*This Woman's Work* by Kate Bush wouldn't work for the meditations, but it was so reflective of the scope of my situation I popped it in anyway. My mind hit rewind, back to those psychic fairs and the hella-accurate astrological birth chart that made a supernatural believer out of me.

I continually plucked gems from it to nurture my inner environment and gain insight into the driving forces behind my behavior.

My mind recalled snippets of *Be Here Now* with its mindfulness teachings and philosophy of self-determination.

*The Road Less Traveled*—'There's a natural inclination to... cling to the old maps and old ways of doing things, to take the easy path.' *The Little Prince's* lessons of 'don't be too concerned with numbers,' and 'find your star,' and his admonishment of the lack of imagination that accompanied adulthood.

Every realization was a spark; every outdated belief, kindling for the pyre.

The Fish Doctor's rejection spoke again: *You're not a candidate for surgery.*

I thought about the satchel of crystals that once hung around Dad's neck, activating his inner healing forces, now dangling from my rearview mirror hopefully doing the same—or at least connecting me to him.

In that moment I realized I'd come further in my healing quest than I gave myself credit for, and I wasn't as alone as I thought. Dad hadn't given me what I wanted, hadn't been there as much as I longed and begged for, I doubted I'd be on the precipice of remission, sparked by a visit from the divine in the hospital, and strengthened by the mind-body connection without him opening the door to the realm beyond the physical.

He set me on the path I was heavily treading. Would I have tapped into and trusted the healing power of my spirit without it? Without him?

I let Kate Bush croon and went to the window to gaze at the almost full moon, continuing to recalibrate from the victim stance of '*Why me?*' to the power position of '*What can I learn from this?*'

In *Love, Medicine & Miracles*, Dr. Siegel said he can often suggest exactly what patients' emotional troubles are, based on the symptoms and location of their disease. After an emergency surgery to remove several feet of dead intestine, one patient said, 'I couldn't handle all the shit that was coming up, or digest the crap in my life.'

My hungry eyes searched the cardboard insert of Louise Hay's general, garden-variety meditation tape case for more.

A week later, two cassettes arrived: *Surgery I & Surgery II* (no flowery titles there). *Surgery I* had a day side with cognitive stretching exercises to expand my mind and positive affirmations to remind me I deserved healing. The B-side played only soft instrumentals so my less-inhibited subconscious could marinade in them while I slept. *Surgery II* was to be played during the operation.

I pictured how it would feel to be well. The energy I'd have, fitting into my regular-sized clothes, having a normal appetite, getting a good night's rest.

Meditations rippled into mindfulness, taking the show on the road. I'd heard an anecdote about Prince telling his band to 'cut themselves in half' (referring to their inner speed) whenever the frenzied energy of performing before massive crowds threatened to sweep them away.

Instead of thinking of my breath as automatic, I thought of it as the stick shift in my AMC Hornet. Mindfulness became a way to drop gears so I could drop into the calm clarity of my center even as the rest of life whizzed by.

I became fully present in everything I did—folding laundry, stirring a cup of coffee, pumping gas—the smallest task was an opportunity to breathe deeply into the mundane. Turning inward and checking on myself took the intensity out of my emotional sails.

Bathrooms became ashrams. I closed my eyes and practiced sinking into my mind, letting go every kind of interference or intrusion by slipping quietly by them.

If treatment for Crohn's was like playing roulette, this statement was the number with *all* my money on it: *The fact that the mind rules the body is, in spite of its neglect by biology and medicine, the most fundamental fact which we know about the process of life.* (Franz Alexander, M.D.).

Graduation night in The Nurturing Program was always bittersweet. The sadness of saying goodbye laced with the sweet satisfaction of helping a family heal their hurtful past. My heart swelled with pride as I watched the families and facilitators celebrate.

I'd benefitted from the healing I facilitated.

Being a program based on honesty, the participants knew what I was going through and what I was going to do about it. They secretly signed a banner to hang on the wall of my hospital room. 'GET WELL SOON!!' in big and bold black, with personal messages of appreciation, hope, and encouragement sprinkled all around.

*I liked listening to you read the meditation lying on the floor in the dark.*

*I hope this surgery fixes you. You're too nice to be sick.*

*Get well quickly so you can help more families like ours.*

I teared up as the unexpected warmth of being seen and valued engulfed me. Instead of brushing it off, I let all their love sink in to support and accompany me.

I checked into the hospital armed with the second meditation tape and that banner.

"Play this while I'm out." I handed the puzzled anesthesiologist *Surgery II*.

As he left to locate a boombox, I turned to my surgeon. (If he was wearing anything fishy under his scrubs, I couldn't tell). "Look, you're going to have direct access to my unconscious in there. Whatever you say goes right in. I can't filter it. So say only good things. Tell me how healthy I look, how strong I am—regardless of what you see. If you must say something negative, you'll have to leave the room first."

His eyes said he still thought I was pretty weird but his nod, making the paper mask scratch against his paper gown, said he would honor my wishes. And while I was jealous of those who had Bernie Siegel as their surgeon, spearheading their healing mindset, I was grateful that mine at least tagged along.

What mattered most was that I believed it. Medical science didn't have all the answers and I'd suffered from that, but failures were just fuel for my journey to find my own way.

"Count backward from ten." The anesthesiologist, back with the boombox, directed.

*I just want to feel good again. I just want to feel good again.*

---

**Core Theme / Emotional Wound:** *Grief + Worthiness.* The point where loss is no longer something to brace against—it's something you *enter* to transmute. The wound shifts from being only about physical pain to the ache of feeling unworthy. Striving to prove your value, and navigating life through performance.

It's also about letting go of the shame that comes from not getting better.

**Old Survival Pattern:** *Self-erasure.* Earning love, proving value, and controlling outcomes. But now, you're replacing control with presence. Instead of chasing, you're letting love *land.* You're finally *receiving* love—even from yourself.

**Gut Instincts Healing Method Stage:** *Free.* This is the *integration* chapter. It's where every little piece you've gathered along the way—the beliefs, the affirmations, meditations, self-inquiry, the losses—begins to cohere. You're not striving anymore. You're *preparing to receive* the next phase of your life with grace and groundedness. You're not just healing symptoms anymore—you're healing your sense of self.

**Reflection:**
This wasn't just about prepping for surgery—it was ceremonial. A sacred rite of passage called self-honoring. Sometimes healing doesn't look like recovery—it seems like surrender.

What if this work—*this woman's work*—isn't about trying harder, but about letting the love in and the healing happen? What if the *work* is to understand our *worth?*

**Reader Reflection:**

1. **Self-Worth and Personal Transformation.** Reflect on a time when you had to move past a limiting belief or external validation to discover your true worth. How did you begin to see yourself differently? Self-worth isn't about earning or proving. It's an inherent truth. Reflect on what shifts you've noticed in your life as you begin to embrace this idea. How does it change the way you make decisions or care for yourself?
2. **Grief and Growth.** Consider a loss that shaped you—not just through pain, but through what it taught you about love, presence, or healing. Grief is more than loss. It's all that love with nowhere to go. It's an invitation to a spiritual relationship. How has grief opened your heart? What gifts or insights has it quietly offered you?
3. **Integration and Receiving.** You've done the work. You've gathered tools, truths, and courage. Now reflect: are you allowing yourself to receive the heal-

ing you've prepared for? How do you let support *land* in your life—emotionally, physically, spiritually? What would it look like to soften your grip and trust the groundwork you've laid?

4. **Mindfulness as Medicine.** Think about the smallest moment today when you slowed down—even for a breath. Did you feel more grounded, more aware, more *here*?

   Mindfulness isn't about silence or stillness. It's about presence. Where in your daily rhythm could you practice being more present?

## Affirmation:

*I am inherently worthy, and my healing is a reflection of my deep trust in myself. I am enough just as I am.*

Scan the Code Below to View the Video for Chapter 29: Or go to: https://youtu.be/kflKidOddWk

## Chapter 30

# Times Like These

**When Inner Knowing Becomes Unshakeable**
Sovereignty, self-trust, and stepping fully into your power.

*I am not what happened to me,*
*I am what I choose to become.*
*~Carl Jung*

The world blurred back into focus. My mother jumped up from her visitor recliner, softly stroking my arm and detailing the morphine drip clicking comfort into my veins. She beamed at me like I imagined she did when they placed me in her arms after making my debut in the world. I faded back into slumber remembering that smile in photos—at my first birthday party smeared into my barely-there hair.

I woke up to her fluffing my pillows, drifting back into dreamland as she tucked me in. My eyes opened to painted nails, then grew heavy as I slipped into sleep, away from such a foreign sight.

She waved away the nurse and while grabbing the sponge and tub from her. "You don't need to bathe her. I'll do that."

The next time I awoke, the Fish Doctor stood by my bed saying I'd looked worse inside than he prepared for. "I had to leave the room and call another surgeon to consult about how much bowel to remove. I didn't want to take too much."

The next day, that second surgeon stood proudly beside him on rounds and pointed to the tape holding my incision shut. "You've got the new Steri-Strips. No dots on the side of your scar from staples, making it look like a caterpillar."

Then, maybe to make his point, he grabbed the corner of the lowest strip and pulled.

We all watched as my skin split open and blood poured out.

Morphine made the scene surreal, but the gasp, the apologetic eyes of my Fish Doctor, and the silence that followed told me it was real. Brain too stunned and body too heavy, I couldn't force the *what the fuck* out of my mouth.

"Guess it's not quite ready," the older surgeon muttered and coughed, changing the subject.

The morphine drip clicked again, luring me back into its cloudy embrace.

With more lucidity came more clarity, so when Josh asked again the next day what he could bring me from home, I answered without even thinking. "My typewriter. I need to update my resume."

Suddenly my job felt too administrative, with too many meetings *talking* about helping people, and not enough time spent actually helping them. The Nurturing Program had the most impact and gave me the most joy, but was less than half my work week. I wanted it to be all of it.

Josh blinked. "But. . . we just bought a house and you got a new car. Your job pays well, the benefits covered this surgery." Sensible thoughts from a sensible man.

I blinked back. Benefits funded my treatment, but belief made it an option to begin with. Josh didn't understand when I tried explaining the inspiration I received as a broadcast from an inner tower that didn't always make sense but I'd learn to trust. Like vowing never to return to that support group. Like knowing surgery was my way out of the bowels of hell.

Six healthy months stretched out before me, granting me permission to pursue my purpose. The more the morphine fog lifted the clearer my vision—to help others the same way I'd helped myself. I didn't want to waste a minute.

Different things mattered—or maybe they were the same things, but they mattered more.

The man who'd been my steady companion in sickness felt farther away as I advanced toward wellness. I'd latched onto the loyalty he offered and my inner child longed for. I'd hidden in him from the self-doubts that shook my sense of self, brushing my broken pieces under the rug.

Was it a relationship or a reprieve?

Our dynamic had always been intermittent. Josh's second-shift schedule meant I came home to an empty house, and he came home to me asleep. We really only saw each other on weekends.

Trees were growing up between our lanes. I'd catch glimpses of him in the gaps between. My inner landscape was also changing. Every step I took toward the supernatural was a step away from us. He didn't want to go in that direction, so I arced further and further from him.

Tap, tap, tap. Drip, drip, drip. Typewriter on my tray table, tubes in my arm like marionette strings. I felt re-missioned before I was even in remission.

In a masterstroke of divine timing, our German Shepherd mix Kaluha gave birth while I was in the hospital. The puppies were growing alongside my healing journey—both of which required patience and rest.

I'd pick a different one before each nap, wrapping a washcloth around their bottom like a diaper, then easing onto the couch as it nuzzled my neck. I nodded off into puppy-breath-scented sleep and dreamt of a calendar without dosage numbers, a full night's sleep, and drinking a real milkshake instead of a medical one.

The puppies were starting new lives and in a way, so was I. A life without pain spiking like a live wire. A life not defined by ER trips or the looming fear of losing control of my bowels. Our wedding was three months away. I wanted my "something new" to be a body that no longer attacked itself.

But the biggest shift was already happening, inside.

Insights into my childhood and my body's breakdown wobbled my foundation. I began to question the person I'd always thought I was. Maybe striving to be the best wasn't the best way to live. The puppies taught me to trust slow growth. Witnessing their steady evolution allowed me to trust mine.

It was the stillest I'd ever been—and for the longest.

Recovery pushed the pause button. All my intentions streamlined into one: *whatever I need to do to support my remission.* Intentions crystallized into revelations. Nobody knew my body better than I did.

When Lori came over to visit, I complained that my pain meds weren't cutting it. She offered me one of hers from the stash in her purse. It gave me better relief, so I called The Fish Doctor's nurse and asked to switch. She obliged but was surprised because my pills were technically stronger.

My body told a different story.

That was the moment it all shifted. Professionals and practitioners could consult, theorize, prescribe—but I was the only one would ever truly know what was right for me.

> *I don't wanna come back down from this cloud.*
> *It's taken me all this time to find out what I need.*
> ~Bush, Comedown

# GUT INSTINCTS

**Core Theme / Emotional Wound:** *Borrowed wholeness + Violation of trust.* This is the "reclaiming" chapter—we are no longer living in reaction to external events, but by our inner compass. It's the healing of self-doubt, and the wound of being dismissed or overruled by "experts." But deeper still, it's the ache of separation from self. From instinct. From ur truth. This chapter begins to mend that rupture.

**Old Survival Pattern:** *Waiting for permission.* You've been checking in with doctors, institutions, even loved ones—always wondering. . . *Is this right? Is it safe? Will this fix my problem? Can I trust the knowing that lives inside me?* But in this chapter, that pattern cracks. A more embodied leadership emerges. Not forceful, but fiercely clear.

**Gut Instincts Healing Method Stage:** *Free.* This is the liberation chapter. You are no longer trying to manage—you are integrating and emerging, aligning your outer world with your inner knowing. You're not "waiting for a solution anymore—you are the solution.

**Reflection:**
I'm still amazed at how quickly I moved from surgical recovery to spiritual revolution. My soul didn't wait for my body, it led from that quiet voice inside—the one that always knows. The one I used to second-guess.

What if your return to self isn't a comeback—it's a becoming? What if radical healing doesn't mean going back to the way things were, but walking forward with a more accurate compass? The same body, maybe—but a whole new True North.

**Reader Reflection:**

1. **Inner Knowing & Bold Choices.** Recall a time you followed your intuition—even when it didn't "make sense" to others. How did that moment shape you? What's one area of your life where you've been waiting for permission? Who gave you the idea that you needed it?
2. **Emergence & Empowerment.** How are you different from the version of yourself that first got sick (or lost, or stuck)? What new identity is emerging for you—one that illness or trauma tried to bury?
3. **Healing as Becoming.** Think about a time when healing asked you to grow—not just feel better, but become someone new. What part of your identity shifted in the process? Who are you becoming?
4. **Inner Authority.** Recall a moment when you knew something about your body or path before anyone else did. What did it feel like to trust that knowing? What makes it easier or harder to trust yourself now?
5. **Letting Go to Grow.** Healing often means outgrowing parts of our past—relationships, roles, or beliefs. Where are you being invited to release something or someone... not in bitterness, but in gratitude?

## Affirmation:

*I trust my body's wisdom.
I am my own best advocate.
Healing is mine to claim.*

# GUT INSTINCTS

Scan the Code Below to View the Video for Chapter 30:
Or go to: https://youtu.be/vi1NM6rVyH8

By the end of Part Three you will recognize patterns and symptoms as messages, reconnect with your inner wisdom, and reclaim complete authority over your life.

# Epilogue

# Best of You

### From Surviving to Thriving
Trauma turned into a self-healing superpower.

*I'm the Phoenix and the ash.*
~Dessa

I sent The Fish Doctor an anniversary card one year after the surgery. And the year after that. And the year after that. To celebrate not just my remission, but the partnership that made it possible—my body and his degree.

That's how all treatment should be. It's how I operate still, thirty-some years later. No blind obedience to white coats and stethoscopes here. I know my body best. After studying it so well for so long, I've got a PhD in Me. I consult practitioners, experts in the field, and even the latest fad—but ultimately I go with my gut. Not just with health decisions, with everything.

Josh and I didn't get married. It's hard to believe someone is Mr. Right when you got with them for the wrong reasons. The more inner work I did, the more my shape shifted until our puzzle pieces no longer fit. It wasn't something I could explain and I'm not sure he would've understood anyway.

My disease may have taken up residency in my digestive system, but it was born from trauma. When I stopped running from the effects of my dysfunctional childhood and reclaimed the parts of me that I'd abandoned, I found myself on sacred ground.

The very patterns that once helped me survive got rinsed clean, transmuting into tools for healing.

- Fierce independence taught me to hear my voice
- Skepticism honed my discernment
- Isolation carved a path to inner connection
- My great need for affection sparked a self-love movement
- From rebel to revolutionary
- Hypervigilance became advocacy

Advocacy that doesn't bulldoze, but *inquires*. That doesn't panic, but *prepares*.

My sensitivity, treated as a negative by my family, ended up saving me. When you trust yourself, you don't need symptoms to speak in all caps. Early awareness is less painful, less disruptive, and way more empowering.

A nurse practitioner of integrative medicine put it like this: The body is a communication device. It starts with a whisper, and it gets louder and louder till you hear it. It'll scream if it has to.

That's what healing gives you—space. Space between stimulus and response. Between the trigger and the spiral. Between the flare-up and the full collapse.

Space to choose differently. That's where your power lives.

Crohn's forced clarity. Louise Hay was right—I could heal my whole life. My disease *had* symptoms, but it also *was* a symptom of my entire ecosystem. That's why medicine failed. Most doctors only looked at the part of me presenting, carving it out and disregarding the rest, seeing the body as separate from the mind.

Just like the old social work model of treating the "problem child" without ever addressing their family or social environment. And just as ineffective.

I view symptoms as the body's love language. An invitation to start unpacking. Gently. Intuitively. Powerfully.

Crohn's did what no accolade or achievement ever could—taught me how to love myself. It showed me that my value doesn't depend on proving, producing, or performing. And that's what finally set me free.

Much like the Japanese art of golden joinery called Kintsugi, my broken pieces were highlighted instead of hidden. The idea that breaks and repairs become part of the beauty, that wholeness includes the cracks filled with gold. That's precisely what the journey is all about—radical healing as wholeness, not erasing what happened.

That's what we are. Gold-lined. Cracked open and made stronger by our mending.

Sometimes I catch a glimpse of the bulb at the base of my scar. It doesn't look like a caterpillar—the old surgeon was right about that. More like a thermometer.

Have you heard the parable?

St. Peter greets a man at Heaven's gate, "Show me your scars."

"I don't have any."

"What a shame." St. Peter replies. "Was there nothing worth fighting for?"

It's hard to believe my fight started with a slip of paper from a nurse. With Dr. Cute & Confident in the doorframe, telling me there were two types of patients.

Now I pass that power on to you.

There is a place in you where nothing is impossible. Consult it. Trust it.

Healing isn't about going back to how you used to be—but forward into more of who you really are. It's evolution, not erasure.

I'm a world traveler now—no longer chained to a toilet or even my country. My freedom rippling to Panama, New Zealand, Europe, Southeast Asia...

I clung to a skiff jumping waves to get to an island off Nicaragua.

But those are stories for the next book.

**Reader Reflection:**

1. **Self-Healing as Reclamation.** Reflect on a part of your story that once brought shame or pain. How might that wound contain wisdom? What have you survived that could be reimagined as strength? What parts of you are asking not just to be fixed—but reclaimed?
2. **From Defense to Power.** Think about a pattern or behavior you've carried for protection—hypervigilance, perfectionism, people-pleasing. What would it look like if you transformed that defense into a self-healing superpower? Can you name its sacred root? Its hidden gift?
3. **You Are the Author.** If someone handed you the pen to write the next chapter of your life, what would the opening line be? What title would your next chapter have? Who do you want to be—not just despite your story, but because of it?

GUT INSTINCTS

## **Affirmation:**

*I trust my inner wisdom
and open myself to the possibility of total healing.
I alone choose what to believe.*

Scan the Code Below to View the Video for the Epilogue:
Or go to: https://youtu.be/WZMT6z0h97Y

## About the Author

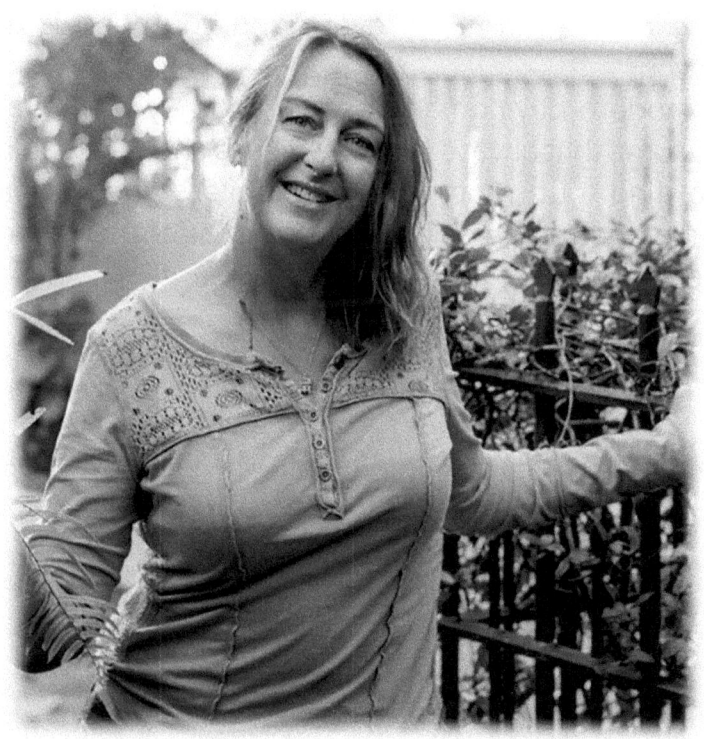

Jennifer Juniper is an international speaker and transformation coach for self-aware women. As the founder of The Inner Compass Collective, she guides them through tailored trans-formational journeys to reclaim their worth, rewire their mind, and rise into their inner authority.

She's on a mission to help the spiritually curious break through the invisible scripts keeping them from the lives they're truly meant to live—unlocking new levels of flow, fulfillment, and freedom.

Through a 12-year immersion in mind-body-spirit practices, Jennifer has spent decades weaving wisdom from quantum physics, psychology, neuroscience, and ancient spiritual teachings into accessible practices.

Known for her grounded yet catalytic presence, Jennifer teaches one radical truth: everything you need is already within you.

A modern-day nomad, Jennifer finds joy in spontaneous adven-tures that always land her where she needs to be.

To find out more about Jennifer's Inner Compass Collective, or to inquire about hiring her as a speaker, you can contact her at:

Email: jen@jenjuniper.com
Website: jenjuniper.com

# Acknowledgements

For this writer, the world is a muse. Everyone I meet shapes me and activates my art in some way. I am grateful to them all, but some gave gifts that made *Gut Instincts* a reality.

To Amber Nolan, without whom this book might never have been written. She helped me see the need for it and kept me company in the process with humor, unbridled honesty (she's from New York), and a periodic kick in the pants (again, New York).

To my Guillotine Girls—Kristina Neihouse, Jessica Argyle, and Josie Mintz—a badass girl writing group dream come true. Without their Sunday afternoon dedication and insights, this book wouldn't be nearly as good.

To Michael Ploof for agitating me in the best of ways by constantly asking me how the writing was going, and to Melanie Ploof for her naturally nurturing presence and spunk—both were infinite sources of motivation.

To my editor, Dr. Linda Sandel Pettit, whose quiet force of belief anchored me when I doubted my voice and gave me the confidence to keep writing.

# JENNIFER JUNIPER

To my publisher, Becky Norwood and Spotlight Publishing House, for her steady support and wisdom—a masterful midwife in the process of birthing a book into the world.

To Victor Jackson, who supports me in everything I do, but especially my writing.

To Joey, I never got his last name, the first person I ever expressed the idea of writing a book to out loud who listened eagerly as I tested my material. His, "You *should* write a book," was the ignition switch.

To Cara Chell who didn't take my "I write when I feel inspired" for an answer. "Writers write," she retorted, and my discipline was born.

To every coffee shop, hotel lobby, bar, café, backseat, bathroom and cocktail napkin that held space for my creative process.

This book was make possible in part, by a grant from the Anne McKee Artists Fund.

We did it!!!

## Did this book speak to you?

I'd love to hear your thoughts!
Your honest review—even a sentence or two—helps
other seekers find this book when they need it most.

www.ingramcontent.com/pod-product-compliance
Lightning Source LLC
Chambersburg PA
CBHW071650090426
42738CB00009B/1481